**PREFACE**

Welcome to "Cure Depression Now." In the modern world, where the pace of life seems to accelerate continually, many individuals find themselves grappling with mental health challenges, with depression being a prevalent and impactful condition. This book is born out of a profound commitment to bring about positive change in the lives of those affected by depression.

## The Motivation Behind the Book

Depression is not just a clinical diagnosis; it's a complex and multifaceted experience that affects individuals on various levels – emotionally, mentally, and physically. The motivation behind this book is rooted in the belief that everyone deserves a chance at a life free from the shackles of depression. It's a call to action, an invitation to embark on a journey toward well-being.

## Navigating the Book

"Cure Depression Now" is not a one-size-fits-all solution. Instead, it's a comprehensive guide that combines scientifically backed methodologies, practical strategies, and holistic approaches to address the diverse aspects of depression. The content is organized to provide a structured pathway for readers, allowing them to navigate through different sections based on their needs and preferences.

## What to Expect

This book covers a wide array of topics, from understanding the nuances of depression to exploring therapeutic techniques, lifestyle adjustments, and fostering resilience. Each chapter is designed to empower readers with knowledge, practical tools, and a sense of hope.

## A Holistic Approach

Recognizing the interconnectedness of mental, emotional, and physical well-being, "Cure Depression Now" adopts a holistic approach. It delves into mindfulness practices, cognitive-behavioral strategies, medication and psychiatry insights, goal-setting techniques, and creative therapies. The aim is to provide a well-rounded toolkit for individuals to reclaim their lives.

## How to Use This Book

Whether you are personally navigating the challenges of depression, supporting a loved one, or a mental health professional seeking additional resources, this book is designed to be accessible and practical. Each section is presented in a concise and reader-friendly manner, encouraging an easy assimilation of information.

## The Path Forward

As you embark on this journey through the pages of "Cure Depression Now," remember that healing is a gradual process. It requires patience, self-compassion, and a commitment to positive change. This book is not a magic cure, but rather a guide that empowers you to take proactive steps toward a brighter, healthier future.

## Join the Conversation

I invite you to join the conversation around mental health and depression. Share your thoughts, experiences, and insights with the community. Let us collectively work towards a world where mental well-being is prioritized, stigma is dismantled, and every individual has the opportunity to thrive.

Thank you for choosing "Cure Depression Now" as part of your journey. Together, let's move towards a future where the shadows of depression are replaced by the warmth of hope.

**N.B. Singh**

# Chapter 1

# Introduction

## 1.1 Understanding Depression

Understanding depression involves recognizing the interplay of various factors that contribute to mental well-being. Let's break it down:

$$\text{Depression} = \text{Biological Factors} + \text{Environmental Stressors} + \text{Cognitive Patterns} \tag{1.1}$$

**Biological Factors:** Genetics $(G)$ and neurochemistry $(N)$ play a crucial role.

$$\text{Biological Factors} = G + N \tag{1.2}$$

**Environmental Stressors:** External influences $(E)$ contribute significantly.

$$\text{Environmental Stressors} = E \tag{1.3}$$

**Cognitive Patterns:** Thoughts $(T)$ and perceptions $(P)$ shape mental states.

$$\text{Cognitive Patterns} = T + P \tag{1.4}$$

Addressing depression involves finding a balance in these components:

$$\text{Balanced Well-being} = \text{Biological Harmony} + \text{Stress Resilience} + \text{Cognitive Equilibrium} \tag{1.5}$$

**Biological Harmony:** Optimal functioning of genetics and neurochemistry.

$$\text{Biological Harmony} = \frac{G}{G_{\text{optimal}}} + \frac{N}{N_{\text{optimal}}} \tag{1.6}$$

**Stress Resilience:** Building resistance to environmental stressors.

$$\text{Stress Resilience} = 1 - \frac{E}{E_{\text{max}}} \tag{1.7}$$

**Cognitive Equilibrium:** Maintaining healthy thought patterns.

$$\text{Cognitive Equilibrium} = \frac{T}{T_{\text{positive}}} + \frac{P}{P_{\text{balanced}}} \tag{1.8}$$

This simplified equation underscores the holistic approach to understanding and addressing depression, emphasizing the need to balance biological, environmental, and cognitive factors.

## 1.2  The Impact of Depression

The impact of depression on an individual's life can be profound and multi-faceted. Let's express it through a mathematical lens:

$$\text{Impact of Depression} = \text{Function}(B, R, S) \tag{1.9}$$

**Biological Disruption ($B$):** Depression can disrupt biological processes, affecting physical health.

$$B = \frac{\text{Genetic Vulnerability} \times \text{Neurochemical Imbalance}}{\text{Optimal Conditions}} \tag{1.10}$$

**Relational Strain ($R$):** Depression often strains relationships, influencing social well-being.

$$R = \frac{\text{Interpersonal Conflicts} \times \text{Emotional Withdrawal}}{\text{Healthy Connection}} \tag{1.11}$$

**Self-Esteem Erosion ($S$):** Depression can erode self-esteem, impacting one's sense of identity.

$$S = \frac{\text{Negative Self-talk} \times \text{Reduced Self-Worth}}{\text{Positive Self-Image}} \tag{1.12}$$

Understanding the impact of depression involves recognizing these factors and their complex interactions:

$$\text{Total Impact} = B + R + S \tag{1.13}$$

Addressing depression requires mitigating these impacts through targeted interventions:

$$\text{Interventions} = \text{Therapy} + \text{Medication} + \text{Support Systems} \tag{1.14}$$

This mathematical representation illustrates the interconnected nature of the impact of depression and the holistic approach needed for effective intervention.

## 1.3 Treatment Options Overview

Navigating treatment options for depression involves understanding the synergistic effects of various approaches. Let's break it down:

$$\text{Treatment Effectiveness} = \text{Therapy} + \text{Medication} + \text{Lifestyle Changes} \tag{1.15}$$

**Therapy** $(T)$**:** Psychotherapy plays a crucial role in addressing cognitive patterns and emotional well-being.

$$T = \frac{\text{Cognitive Restructuring} + \text{Behavioral Activation}}{\text{Sessions Attended}} \tag{1.16}$$

**Medication** $(M)$**:** Pharmacological interventions aim to restore neurochemical balance.

$$M = \frac{\text{Selective Serotonin Reuptake Inhibitors (SSRIs)} + \text{Neurotransmitter Modulation}}{\text{Dosage Compliance}} \tag{1.17}$$

**Lifestyle Changes** $(L)$**:** Adopting a healthy lifestyle contributes to overall well-being.

$$L = \frac{\text{Regular Exercise} + \text{Balanced Nutrition}}{\text{Consistency}} \tag{1.18}$$

The holistic impact of treatment options is a combined effort:

$$\text{Total Treatment Impact} = T + M + L \tag{1.19}$$

Additionally, let's represent the concept of synergy in treatment:

$$\text{Synergy} = \text{Therapy} \times \text{Medication} \times \text{Lifestyle Changes} \tag{1.20}$$

This formula emphasizes the enhanced effectiveness when therapy, medication, and lifestyle changes work together synergistically.

Understanding these equations provides a framework for individuals and professionals to optimize treatment plans tailored to each person's unique needs.

## 1.4 Setting the Foundation for Recovery

Establishing a strong foundation for recovery involves key elements that can be expressed mathematically. Let's explore:

$$\text{Foundation Strength} = \text{Self-Care} + \text{Resilience} + \text{Support Systems} \tag{1.21}$$

**Self-Care** $(S)$**:** Prioritizing personal well-being is fundamental to recovery.

$$S = \frac{\text{Healthy Habits} + \text{Mindful Practices}}{\text{Consistency}} \tag{1.22}$$

**Resilience ($R$):** Building resilience is essential for navigating challenges.

$$R = \frac{\text{Adaptability} + \text{Positive Mindset}}{\text{Coping Strategies}} \tag{1.23}$$

**Support Systems ($SS$):** Having a strong support network contributes significantly.

$$SS = \frac{\text{Family Support} + \text{Friendships} + \text{Professional Guidance}}{\text{Quality of Relationships}} \tag{1.24}$$

The synergy of these components forms the bedrock for recovery:

$$\text{Total Foundation} = S + R + SS \tag{1.25}$$

To emphasize the interconnected nature of self-care, resilience, and support systems:

$$\text{Interconnectedness} = \text{Self-Care} \times \text{Resilience} \times \text{Support Systems} \tag{1.26}$$

This formula highlights the holistic approach to setting a robust foundation for recovery.

Understanding these equations empowers individuals to actively contribute to their recovery journey by focusing on these foundational elements.

## 1.5　The Importance of Seeking Help

Recognizing the value of seeking help for mental health can be expressed through mathematical insights. Let's delve into the equations:

$$\text{Benefits of Help} = \text{Professional Support} + \text{Community Resources} + \text{Personal Growth} \tag{1.27}$$

**Professional Support ($PS$):** Engaging with mental health professionals is a cornerstone of seeking help.

$$PS = \frac{\text{Therapist Expertise} + \text{Psychiatrist Guidance}}{\text{Session Consistency}} \tag{1.28}$$

**Community Resources ($CR$):** Utilizing community resources enhances the support network.

$$CR = \frac{\text{Support Groups} + \text{Helplines}}{\text{Active Participation}} \tag{1.29}$$

**Personal Growth ($PG$):** Seeking help contributes to personal development.

$$PG = \frac{\text{Self-Discovery} + \text{Resilience Building}}{\text{Commitment to Growth}} \tag{1.30}$$

The cumulative effect of these elements emphasizes the importance of seeking help:

$$\text{Total Importance} = PS + CR + PG \tag{1.31}$$

Additionally, let's represent the concept of empowerment through seeking help:

$$\text{Empowerment} = \text{Professional Support} \times \text{Community Resources} \times \text{Personal Growth} \tag{1.32}$$

This formula underscores the empowering impact when professional support, community resources, and personal growth work together.

Understanding these equations provides a framework for individuals to appreciate the transformative power of seeking help for their mental well-being.

## 1.6 Breaking the Stigma

The process of breaking the stigma surrounding mental health can be expressed through mathematical insights. Let's explore:

$$\text{Stigma Reduction} = \text{Education} + \text{Open Conversations} + \text{Empathy} \tag{1.33}$$

**Education ($E$):** Increasing knowledge about mental health is key to breaking the stigma.

$$E = \frac{\text{Awareness Programs} + \text{Media Literacy}}{\text{Information Dissemination}} \tag{1.34}$$

**Open Conversations ($OC$):** Encouraging dialogue fosters understanding and acceptance.

$$OC = \frac{\text{Personal Stories} + \text{Media Representation}}{\text{Conversation Accessibility}} \tag{1.35}$$

**Empathy ($EM$):** Cultivating empathy helps break down judgment and prejudice.

$$EM = \frac{\text{Perspective-Taking} + \text{Non-judgmental Attitude}}{\text{Compassion Development}} \tag{1.36}$$

The holistic impact of these components contributes to breaking the stigma:

$$\text{Total Stigma Breakage} = E + OC + EM \tag{1.37}$$

Additionally, let's represent the idea of societal transformation through stigma reduction:

$$\text{Societal Transformation} = \text{Education} \times \text{Open Conversations} \times \text{Empathy} \tag{1.38}$$

This formula highlights the collective power of education, open conversations, and empathy in transforming societal perspectives.

Understanding these equations provides a framework for individuals and communities to actively participate in breaking the stigma surrounding mental health.

## 1.7 Embarking on Your Recovery Journey

Embarking on a recovery journey involves dynamic elements that can be expressed through mathematical insights. Let's delve into the equations:

$$\text{Recovery Progress} = \text{Commitment} + \text{Adaptability} + \text{Positive Choices} \tag{1.39}$$

**Commitment** ($C$): A strong commitment is the foundation of a successful recovery journey.

$$C = \frac{\text{Goal Setting} + \text{Consistency}}{\text{Personal Dedication}} \tag{1.40}$$

**Adaptability** ($A$): Being adaptable allows for flexibility in navigating challenges.

$$A = \frac{\text{Resilience} + \text{Learning from Setbacks}}{\text{Open-mindedness}} \tag{1.41}$$

**Positive Choices** ($PC$): Making positive choices contributes to overall well-being.

$$PC = \frac{\text{Healthy Lifestyle} + \text{Mindfulness Practices}}{\text{Intentional Decision-Making}} \tag{1.42}$$

The cumulative effect of these elements symbolizes the journey of recovery:

$$\text{Total Journey} = C + A + PC \tag{1.43}$$

Additionally, let's represent the concept of personal transformation during the recovery journey:

$$\text{Transformation} = \text{Commitment} \times \text{Adaptability} \times \text{Positive Choices} \tag{1.44}$$

This formula emphasizes the transformative power of commitment, adaptability, and positive choices during the recovery process.

Understanding these equations provides individuals with a mathematical framework to actively engage and progress on their unique recovery journey.

# Chapter 2

# Identifying Triggers

## 2.1 Recognizing Personal Triggers

Efficiently recognizing personal triggers involves practical insights that can be expressed through mathematical formulas. Let's explore:

$$\text{Trigger Awareness} = \text{Self-Reflection} + \text{Environmental Factors} + \text{Behavioral Patterns} \tag{2.1}$$

**Self-Reflection** $(SR)$: Deep self-reflection is fundamental to trigger awareness.

$$SR = \frac{\text{Thought Journaling} + \text{Emotional Tracking}}{\text{Consistent Practice}} \tag{2.2}$$

**Environmental Factors** $(EF)$: Identifying external triggers is crucial for proactive management.

$$EF = \frac{\text{Stressful Events} + \text{Social Situations}}{\text{Observational Skills}} \tag{2.3}$$

**Behavioral Patterns** $(BP)$: Recognizing behavioral cues helps pinpoint triggers.

$$BP = \frac{\text{Habitual Reactions} + \text{Response Patterns}}{\text{Behavioral Analysis}} \tag{2.4}$$

The synergy of these components forms the basis for trigger recognition:

$$\text{Total Awareness} = SR + EF + BP \tag{2.5}$$

Additionally, let's represent the idea of trigger identification efficiency:

$$\text{Efficiency} = \text{Self-Reflection} \times \text{Environmental Factors} \times \text{Behavioral Patterns} \tag{2.6}$$

This formula highlights the efficiency gained when self-reflection, environmental factors, and behavioral patterns work together in identifying personal triggers.

Understanding these equations provides individuals with practical tools to efficiently recognize and manage their personal triggers.

## 2.2 External Factors and Their Role

Understanding the impact of external factors on triggers involves practical insights expressed through mathematical formulas. Let's delve into the equations:

$$\text{Trigger Influence} = \text{External Stressors} + \text{Social Environments} + \text{Life Events} \tag{2.7}$$

**External Stressors** ($ES$): Quantifying the influence of external stressors is crucial for trigger management.

$$ES = \frac{\text{Work Pressure} + \text{Financial Stress}}{\text{Stress Intensity}} \tag{2.8}$$

**Social Environments** ($SE$): Assessing the impact of social environments helps identify potential triggers.

$$SE = \frac{\text{Social Expectations} + \text{Peer Influences}}{\text{Social Dynamics}} \tag{2.9}$$

**Life Events** ($LE$): Recognizing the role of significant life events contributes to trigger awareness.

$$LE = \frac{\text{Major Changes} + \text{Losses}}{\text{Life Transition Magnitude}} \tag{2.10}$$

The interconnectedness of these external factors shapes the overall trigger influence:

$$\text{Total Influence} = ES + SE + LE \tag{2.11}$$

Additionally, let's represent the idea of external factor balance:

$$\text{Balance} = \text{External Stressors} \times \text{Social Environments} \times \text{Life Events} \tag{2.12}$$

This formula highlights the importance of maintaining balance among external stressors, social environments, and life events to mitigate trigger impact.

Understanding these equations provides individuals with practical tools to assess and manage the influence of external factors on their triggers.

## 2.3 Coping Strategies

Efficiently employing coping strategies involves practical insights expressed through mathematical formulas. Let's explore:

$$\text{Coping Effectiveness} = \text{Mindfulness} + \text{Positive Distractions} + \text{Emotional Regulation} \quad (2.13)$$

**Mindfulness ($M$):** Cultivating mindfulness is a key element of effective coping.

$$M = \frac{\text{Breathing Exercises} + \text{Meditation}}{\text{Present-Moment Focus}} \quad (2.14)$$

**Positive Distractions ($PD$):** Utilizing positive distractions contributes to coping effectiveness.

$$PD = \frac{\text{Hobbies} + \text{Creative Outlets}}{\text{Engagement Level}} \quad (2.15)$$

**Emotional Regulation ($ER$):** Developing emotional regulation skills is essential for coping.

$$ER = \frac{\text{Identifying Emotions} + \text{Healthy Expression}}{\text{Emotional Balance}} \quad (2.16)$$

The synergistic effect of these coping strategies forms the basis for effective management:

$$\text{Total Effectiveness} = M + PD + ER \quad (2.17)$$

Additionally, let's represent the concept of coping resilience:

$$\text{Resilience} = \text{Mindfulness} \times \text{Positive Distractions} \times \text{Emotional Regulation} \quad (2.18)$$

This formula underscores the resilience gained when mindfulness, positive distractions, and emotional regulation work together in coping with triggers.

Understanding these equations provides individuals with practical tools to efficiently employ coping strategies in their daily lives.

## 2.4 Triggers in Daily Life

Identifying triggers in daily life involves practical insights expressed through mathematical formulas. Let's explore:

$$\text{Daily Trigger Occurrence} = \text{Routine Exposures} + \text{Interpersonal Dynamics} \\ + \text{Environmental Influences} \quad (2.19)$$

**Routine Exposures ($RE$):** Recognizing triggers in daily routines is essential for proactive management.

$$RE = \frac{\text{Work Habits} + \text{Daily Tasks}}{\text{Exposure Frequency}} \tag{2.20}$$

**Interpersonal Dynamics ($ID$):** Understanding triggers in social interactions contributes to awareness.

$$ID = \frac{\text{Communication Patterns} + \text{Relationship Dynamics}}{\text{Interpersonal Sensitivity}} \tag{2.21}$$

**Environmental Influences ($EI$):** Identifying triggers in the surrounding environment is crucial for proactive coping.

$$EI = \frac{\text{Physical Spaces} + \text{Ambient Factors}}{\text{Environmental Awareness}} \tag{2.22}$$

The cumulative effect of these trigger sources shapes the overall trigger occurrence:

$$\text{Total Occurrence} = RE + ID + EI \tag{2.23}$$

Additionally, let's represent the concept of trigger awareness:

$$\text{Awareness} = \text{Routine Exposures} \times \text{Interpersonal Dynamics} \times \text{Environmental Influences} \tag{2.24}$$

This formula underscores the importance of maintaining awareness in routine exposures, interpersonal dynamics, and environmental influences to effectively identify triggers in daily life.

Understanding these equations provides individuals with practical tools to efficiently recognize and manage triggers encountered in their daily routines.

## 2.5   Addressing Triggers Proactively

Proactively addressing triggers involves practical insights expressed through mathematical formulas. Let's delve into the equations:

$$\text{Proactive Response} = \text{Mindfulness} + \text{Strategic Planning} + \text{Behavioral Interventions} \tag{2.25}$$

**Mindfulness ($M$):** Cultivating mindfulness is a key element of a proactive response to triggers.

$$M = \frac{\text{Present-Moment Awareness} + \text{Mindful Breathing}}{\text{Focused Attention}} \tag{2.26}$$

**Strategic Planning ($SP$):** Planning strategies ahead of time enhances proactive response.

$$SP = \frac{\text{Trigger Identification} + \text{Preemptive Actions}}{\text{Strategic Thinking}} \tag{2.27}$$

**Behavioral Interventions ($BI$):** Implementing behavioral interventions is crucial for addressing triggers.

$$BI = \frac{\text{Positive Replacements} + \text{Adaptive Responses}}{\text{Behavioral Modification}} \tag{2.28}$$

The combined effect of these proactive elements forms the basis for addressing triggers proactively:

$$\text{Total Proactivity} = M + SP + BI \tag{2.29}$$

Additionally, let's represent the concept of proactive resilience:

$$\text{Resilience} = \text{Mindfulness} \times \text{Strategic Planning} \times \text{Behavioral Interventions} \tag{2.30}$$

This formula underscores the resilience gained when mindfulness, strategic planning, and behavioral interventions work together in proactively addressing triggers.

Understanding these equations provides individuals with practical tools to efficiently and proactively respond to triggers in their daily lives.

## 2.6 Mind-Body Connections

Understanding mind-body connections in the context of triggers involves practical insights expressed through mathematical formulas. Let's explore:

$$\text{Mind-Body Harmony} = \text{Emotional Awareness} + \text{Physical Well-being} + \text{Cognitive Balance} \tag{2.31}$$

**Emotional Awareness** ($EA$): Being in tune with emotions contributes to mind-body harmony.

$$EA = \frac{\text{Emotion Recognition} + \text{Emotional Expression}}{\text{Emotional Intelligence}} \tag{2.32}$$

**Physical Well-being** ($PW$): Maintaining physical health supports a balanced mind-body connection.

$$PW = \frac{\text{Exercise Regularity} + \text{Nutritional Balance}}{\text{Physical Vitality}} \tag{2.33}$$

**Cognitive Balance** ($CB$): Achieving cognitive balance enhances mind-body connections.

$$CB = \frac{\text{Positive Thinking} + \text{Stress Management}}{\text{Cognitive Equilibrium}} \tag{2.34}$$

The holistic effect of these components forms the basis for mind-body connections:

$$\text{Total Harmony} = EA + PW + CB \tag{2.35}$$

Additionally, let's represent the idea of interconnectedness in mind-body connections:

$$\text{Interconnectedness} = \text{Emotional Awareness} \times \text{Physical Well-being} \times \text{Cognitive Balance} \tag{2.36}$$

This formula highlights the interconnected nature of emotional awareness, physical well-being, and cognitive balance in fostering mind-body harmony.

Understanding these equations provides individuals with practical tools to enhance mind-body connections and navigate triggers more effectively.

## 2.7   Self-Reflection for Personal Growth

Engaging in self-reflection for personal growth involves practical insights expressed through mathematical formulas. Let's explore:

$$\text{Personal Growth Index} = \text{Reflection Depth} + \text{Learning Attitude} + \text{Action Implementation} \tag{2.37}$$

**Reflection Depth ($RD$):** The depth of self-reflection is crucial for personal growth.

$$RD = \frac{\text{Thoughtful Contemplation} + \text{Value Assessment}}{\text{Reflective Depth}} \tag{2.38}$$

**Learning Attitude ($LA$):** Adopting a positive learning attitude enhances personal growth.

$$LA = \frac{\text{Open-mindedness} + \text{Curiosity}}{\text{Learning Enthusiasm}} \tag{2.39}$$

**Action Implementation ($AI$):** Translating insights into action is key for personal growth.

$$AI = \frac{\text{Goal Setting} + \text{Behavioral Changes}}{\text{Action Effectiveness}} \tag{2.40}$$

The combined effect of these elements forms the basis for personal growth through self-reflection:

$$\text{Total Growth} = RD + LA + AI \tag{2.41}$$

Additionally, let's represent the concept of transformative power in personal growth:

$$\text{Transformation} = \text{Reflection Depth} \times \text{Learning Attitude} \times \text{Action Implementation} \tag{2.42}$$

This formula underscores the transformative power of deep reflection, a positive learning attitude, and effective action implementation in fostering personal growth.

Understanding these equations provides individuals with practical tools to engage in self-reflection for continuous personal development.

# Chapter 3

# Holistic Approaches

## 3.1  Mind-Body Connection

Fostering a strong mind-body connection involves practical insights expressed through mathematical formulas. Let's explore:

$$\text{Mind-Body Synergy} = \text{Mental Harmony} + \text{Physical Well-being} + \text{Emotional Equilibrium} \quad (3.1)$$

**Mental Harmony** ($MH$): Achieving mental harmony is crucial for the mind-body connection.

$$MH = \frac{\text{Cognitive Balance} + \text{Stress Management}}{\text{Mental Equanimity}} \quad (3.2)$$

**Physical Well-being** ($PW$): Maintaining physical health contributes to the mind-body connection.

$$PW = \frac{\text{Exercise Regularity} + \text{Nutritional Balance}}{\text{Physical Vitality}} \quad (3.3)$$

**Emotional Equilibrium** ($EE$): Balancing emotions enhances the mind-body connection.

$$EE = \frac{\text{Emotion Recognition} + \text{Emotional Expression}}{\text{Emotional Balance}} \quad (3.4)$$

The combined effect of these components forms the basis for a holistic mind-body connection:

$$\text{Total Synergy} = MH + PW + EE \quad (3.5)$$

Additionally, let's represent the idea of interconnectedness in the mind-body connection:

$$\text{Interconnectedness} = \text{Mental Harmony} \times \text{Physical Well-being} \times \text{Emotional Equilibrium} \quad (3.6)$$

This formula underscores the interconnected nature of mental harmony, physical well-being, and emotional equilibrium in fostering a strong mind-body connection.

Understanding these equations provides individuals with practical tools to enhance the holistic connection between their mind and body.

## 3.2  Nutrition and Mental Health

Understanding the link between nutrition and mental health involves practical insights expressed through mathematical formulas. Let's explore:

$$\text{Mental Health Boost} = \text{Balanced Diet} + \text{Nutrient Absorption} + \text{Hydration Level} \tag{3.7}$$

**Balanced Diet** ($BD$): Consuming a balanced diet is fundamental for mental health.

$$BD = \frac{\text{Essential Nutrients} + \text{Dietary Diversity}}{\text{Nutritional Balance}} \tag{3.8}$$

**Nutrient Absorption** ($NA$): Efficient nutrient absorption enhances mental health benefits.

$$NA = \frac{\text{Gut Health} + \text{Digestive Efficiency}}{\text{Nutrient Assimilation}} \tag{3.9}$$

**Hydration Level** ($HL$): Maintaining proper hydration contributes to mental well-being.

$$HL = \frac{\text{Water Intake} + \text{Hydration Consistency}}{\text{Hydration Balance}} \tag{3.10}$$

The cumulative effect of these nutritional factors forms the basis for a holistic approach to mental health:

$$\text{Total Boost} = BD + NA + HL \tag{3.11}$$

Additionally, let's represent the concept of nutritional synergy:

$$\text{Nutritional Synergy} = \text{Balanced Diet} \times \text{Nutrient Absorption} \times \text{Hydration Level} \tag{3.12}$$

This formula underscores the synergistic nature of a balanced diet, efficient nutrient absorption, and proper hydration in promoting mental health.

Understanding these equations provides individuals with practical tools to leverage nutrition for holistic mental well-being.

## 3.3 Exercise and Well-being

Understanding the connection between exercise and well-being involves practical insights expressed through mathematical formulas. Let's explore:

$$\text{Well-being Enhancement} = \text{Physical Activity} + \text{Endorphin Release} + \text{Consistency Level} \quad (3.13)$$

**Physical Activity** ($PA$)**:** Engaging in regular physical activity is fundamental for well-being.

$$PA = \frac{\text{Cardiovascular Exercise} + \text{Strength Training}}{\text{Physical Engagement}} \quad (3.14)$$

**Endorphin Release** ($ER$)**:** The release of endorphins contributes to the positive effects of exercise.

$$ER = \frac{\text{Duration of Exercise} + \text{Intensity Level}}{\text{Endorphin Response}} \quad (3.15)$$

**Consistency Level** ($CL$)**:** Maintaining consistent exercise habits enhances overall well-being.

$$CL = \frac{\text{Frequency of Exercise} + \text{Routine Stability}}{\text{Consistency Rating}} \quad (3.16)$$

The combined effect of these exercise factors forms the basis for a holistic approach to well-being:

$$\text{Total Enhancement} = PA + ER + CL \quad (3.17)$$

Additionally, let's represent the concept of well-being synergy:

$$\text{Well-being Synergy} = \text{Physical Activity} \times \text{Endorphin Release} \times \text{Consistency Level} \quad (3.18)$$

This formula underscores the synergistic nature of regular physical activity, endorphin release, and consistent exercise in promoting overall well-being.

Understanding these equations provides individuals with practical tools to leverage exercise for holistic well-being.

## 3.4 Alternative Therapies

Exploring alternative therapies for holistic well-being involves practical insights expressed through mathematical formulas. Let's delve into the equations:

$$\text{Holistic Balance} = \text{Mind-Body Alignment} + \text{Energy Flow} + \text{Therapeutic Consistency} \quad (3.19)$$

**Mind-Body Alignment** ($MBA$)**:** Achieving alignment between the mind and body is foundational for holistic balance.

$$MBA = \frac{\text{Mindfulness Practices} + \text{Body-Mind Techniques}}{\text{Holistic Synchronization}} \tag{3.20}$$

**Energy Flow** ($EF$): Enhancing the flow of energy through alternative therapies contributes to holistic well-being.

$$EF = \frac{\text{Qi Gong} + \text{Reiki Practices}}{\text{Energy Harmony}} \tag{3.21}$$

**Therapeutic Consistency** ($TC$): Maintaining consistent engagement in alternative therapies is essential for holistic balance.

$$TC = \frac{\text{Therapy Sessions} + \text{Self-Care Practices}}{\text{Consistency Rating}} \tag{3.22}$$

The holistic effect of these alternative therapy components forms the basis for a well-rounded approach to well-being:

$$\text{Total Holism} = MBA + EF + TC \tag{3.23}$$

Additionally, let's represent the concept of therapeutic synergy:

$$\text{Therapeutic Synergy} = \text{Mind-Body Alignment} \times \text{Energy Flow} \times \text{Therapeutic Consistency} \tag{3.24}$$

This formula underscores the synergistic nature of mind-body alignment, energy flow, and therapeutic consistency in promoting holistic well-being through alternative therapies.

Understanding these equations provides individuals with practical tools to explore and integrate alternative therapies for a comprehensive approach to well-being.

## 3.5　Exploring Holistic Healing

Embarking on the journey of holistic healing involves practical insights expressed through mathematical formulas. Let's delve into the equations:

$$\text{Holistic Harmony} = \text{Body-Mind Alignment} + \text{Energy Equilibrium} + \text{Integrated Practices} \tag{3.25}$$

**Body-Mind Alignment** ($BMA$): Achieving alignment between the body and mind is foundational for holistic harmony.

$$BMA = \frac{\text{Mindfulness Techniques} + \text{Physical Well-being Practices}}{\text{Holistic Synchronization}} \tag{3.26}$$

**Energy Equilibrium** ($EE$): Balancing the flow of energy contributes to overall well-being in holistic healing.

$$EE = \frac{\text{Qi Gong} + \text{Chakra Balancing}}{\text{Energy Harmony}} \quad (3.27)$$

**Integrated Practices** ($IP$): Incorporating diverse holistic practices enhances the holistic healing journey.

$$IP = \frac{\text{Alternative Therapies} + \text{Mind-Body Exercises}}{\text{Integrated Wellness}} \quad (3.28)$$

The combined effect of these holistic components forms the basis for a comprehensive approach to healing:

$$\text{Total Holism} = BMA + EE + IP \quad (3.29)$$

Additionally, let's represent the concept of holistic synergy:

$$\text{Holistic Synergy} = \text{Body-Mind Alignment} \times \text{Energy Equilibrium} \times \text{Integrated Practices} \quad (3.30)$$

This formula underscores the synergistic nature of body-mind alignment, energy equilibrium, and integrated practices in promoting holistic well-being.

Understanding these equations provides individuals with practical tools to explore and embrace holistic healing for a balanced and integrated life.

## 3.6 Integrating Holistic Practices

Creating a harmonious integration of holistic practices involves practical insights expressed through mathematical formulas. Let's delve into the equations:

$$\begin{aligned}
\text{Holistic Integration} = {} &\text{Mind-Body Synergy} + \text{Nutritional Balance} \\
&+ \text{Exercise Harmony} + \text{Therapeutic Synchronization}
\end{aligned} \quad (3.31)$$

**Mind-Body Synergy** ($MBS$): Fostering synergy between the mind and body is foundational for holistic integration.

$$MBS = \frac{\text{Mindfulness} + \text{Physical Well-being}}{\text{Holistic Alignment}} \quad (3.32)$$

**Nutritional Balance** ($NB$): Achieving balance in nutrition contributes to overall well-being in holistic integration.

$$NB = \frac{\text{Balanced Diet} + \text{Nutrient Absorption}}{\text{Nutritional Harmony}} \quad (3.33)$$

**Exercise Harmony** ($EH$): Balancing exercise routines enhances the holistic integration of well-being.

$$EH = \frac{\text{Physical Activity} + \text{Endorphin Release}}{\text{Exercise Equilibrium}} \tag{3.34}$$

**Therapeutic Synchronization ($TS$):** Synchronizing therapeutic practices contributes to the overall integration of holistic well-being.

$$TS = \frac{\text{Alternative Therapies} + \text{Mind-Body Practices}}{\text{Therapeutic Balance}} \tag{3.35}$$

The combined effect of these integrated components forms the basis for a comprehensive approach to holistic living:

$$\text{Total Integration} = MBS + NB + EH + TS \tag{3.36}$$

Additionally, let's represent the concept of holistic synergy:

$$\begin{aligned} \text{Holistic Synergy} = {} & \text{Mind-Body Synergy} \times \text{Nutritional Balance} \\ & \times \text{Exercise Harmony} \times \text{Therapeutic Synchronization} \end{aligned} \tag{3.37}$$

This formula underscores the synergistic nature of mind-body synergy, nutritional balance, exercise harmony, and therapeutic synchronization in promoting holistic well-being through integrated practices.

Understanding these equations provides individuals with practical tools to seamlessly integrate various holistic practices for a balanced and harmonious lifestyle.

## 3.7    Creating a Holistic Lifestyle

Building a holistic lifestyle involves practical insights expressed through mathematical formulas. Let's explore the equations:

$$\begin{aligned} \text{Holistic Living Index} = {} & \text{Mind-Body Synergy} + \text{Nutritional Harmony} \\ & + \text{Exercise Equilibrium} + \text{Therapeutic Balance} \end{aligned} \tag{3.38}$$

**Mind-Body Synergy ($MBS$):** Fostering synergy between the mind and body is foundational for a holistic lifestyle.

$$MBS = \frac{\text{Mindfulness} + \text{Physical Well-being}}{\text{Holistic Alignment}} \tag{3.39}$$

**Nutritional Harmony ($NH$):** Achieving harmony in nutrition contributes to overall well-being in a holistic lifestyle.

$$NH = \frac{\text{Balanced Diet} + \text{Nutrient Absorption}}{\text{Nutritional Equilibrium}} \tag{3.40}$$

**Exercise Equilibrium** ($EE$): Balancing exercise routines enhances the holistic lifestyle.

$$EE = \frac{\text{Physical Activity} + \text{Endorphin Release}}{\text{Exercise Balance}} \tag{3.41}$$

**Therapeutic Balance** ($TB$): Striking a balance in therapeutic practices contributes to the overall harmony of a holistic lifestyle.

$$TB = \frac{\text{Alternative Therapies} + \text{Mind-Body Practices}}{\text{Therapeutic Synergy}} \tag{3.42}$$

The combined effect of these holistic components forms the basis for a comprehensive approach to living holistically:

$$\text{Total Holism} = MBS + NH + EE + TB \tag{3.43}$$

Additionally, let's represent the concept of holistic synergy:

$$\text{Holistic Synergy} = \text{Mind-Body Synergy} \times \text{Nutritional Harmony} \\ \times \text{Exercise Equilibrium} \times \text{Therapeutic Balance} \tag{3.44}$$

This formula underscores the synergistic nature of mind-body synergy, nutritional harmony, exercise equilibrium, and therapeutic balance in creating a holistic lifestyle.

Understanding these equations provides individuals with practical tools to embody and sustain a holistic approach to life.

# Chapter 4

# Building a Support System

## 4.1 Family Dynamics

Understanding and enhancing family dynamics for a strong support system involves practical insights expressed through mathematical formulas. Let's explore:

$$\text{Family Support Index} = \text{Communication Strength} + \text{Emotional Resilience} + \text{Collaborative Harmony} \tag{4.1}$$

**Communication Strength** ($CS$)**:** Fostering strong communication is fundamental for family support.

$$CS = \frac{\text{Open Communication} + \text{Active Listening}}{\text{Communication Effectiveness}} \tag{4.2}$$

**Emotional Resilience** ($ER$)**:** Building emotional resilience within the family contributes to overall support.

$$ER = \frac{\text{Emotion Regulation} + \text{Empathy}}{\text{Emotional Stability}} \tag{4.3}$$

**Collaborative Harmony** ($CH$)**:** Achieving collaborative harmony enhances the support system within the family.

$$CH = \frac{\text{Conflict Resolution} + \text{Shared Responsibilities}}{\text{Collaborative Equilibrium}} \tag{4.4}$$

The combined effect of these family dynamics components forms the basis for a strong and supportive family system:

$$\text{Total Support} = CS + ER + CH \tag{4.5}$$

Additionally, let's represent the idea of family unity:

$$\text{Family Unity} = \text{Communication Strength} \times \text{Emotional Resilience} \times \text{Collaborative Harmony} \quad (4.6)$$

This formula underscores the interconnected nature of communication strength, emotional resilience, and collaborative harmony in building a supportive family system.

Understanding these equations provides families with practical tools to strengthen their dynamics and create a resilient and supportive environment.

## 4.2  Friendships and Social Support

Cultivating strong friendships and social support involves practical insights expressed through mathematical formulas. Let's explore:

$$\text{Social Support Index} = \text{Connection Depth} + \text{Empathetic Network} + \text{Reciprocal Reliability} \quad (4.7)$$

**Connection Depth ($CD$):** Fostering deep connections is fundamental for social support.

$$CD = \frac{\text{Quality Time} + \text{Shared Experiences}}{\text{Connection Intimacy}} \quad (4.8)$$

**Empathetic Network ($EN$):** Building an empathetic social network contributes to overall support.

$$EN = \frac{\text{Understanding} + \text{Supportive Listening}}{\text{Empathy Strength}} \quad (4.9)$$

**Reciprocal Reliability ($RR$):** Establishing reciprocal reliability enhances the support within friendships.

$$RR = \frac{\text{Mutual Assistance} + \text{Reliable Availability}}{\text{Reciprocal Trust}} \quad (4.10)$$

The combined effect of these friendship and social support components forms the basis for a strong and reliable support system:

$$\text{Total Support} = CD + EN + RR \quad (4.11)$$

Additionally, let's represent the concept of social cohesion:

$$\text{Social Cohesion} = \text{Connection Depth} \times \text{Empathetic Network} \times \text{Reciprocal Reliability} \quad (4.12)$$

This formula underscores the synergistic nature of connection depth, empathetic network, and reciprocal reliability in building a supportive social environment.

Understanding these equations provides individuals with practical tools to nurture and strengthen their friendships, creating a robust social support system.

## 4.3  Professional Assistance

Seeking and utilizing professional assistance involves practical insights expressed through mathematical formulas. Let's explore:

$$\text{Professional Support Index} = \text{Expertise Depth} + \text{Collaborative Synergy} + \text{Therapeutic Effectiveness} \tag{4.13}$$

**Expertise Depth ($ED$):** Leveraging the depth of expertise is fundamental for professional support.

$$ED = \frac{\text{Specialized Knowledge} + \text{Experience Mastery}}{\text{Expertise Proficiency}} \tag{4.14}$$

**Collaborative Synergy ($CS$):** Building collaborative synergy enhances the support from professionals.

$$CS = \frac{\text{Team Coordination} + \text{Interdisciplinary Collaboration}}{\text{Collaborative Efficiency}} \tag{4.15}$$

**Therapeutic Effectiveness ($TE$):** Ensuring therapeutic effectiveness contributes to the overall support from professionals.

$$TE = \frac{\text{Intervention Impact} + \text{Client Progress}}{\text{Therapeutic Success}} \tag{4.16}$$

The combined effect of these professional assistance components forms the basis for a strong and effective support system:

$$\text{Total Support} = ED + CS + TE \tag{4.17}$$

Additionally, let's represent the concept of professional collaboration:

$$\text{Professional Collaboration} = \text{Expertise Depth} \times \text{Collaborative Synergy} \times \text{Therapeutic Effectiveness} \tag{4.18}$$

This formula underscores the synergistic nature of expertise depth, collaborative synergy, and therapeutic effectiveness in building a robust professional support system.

Understanding these equations provides individuals with practical tools to navigate and benefit from professional assistance for a comprehensive support network.

## 4.4  Online Communities and Resources

Leveraging online communities and resources for support involves practical insights expressed through mathematical formulas. Let's explore:

$$\text{Digital Support Index} = \text{Community Engagement} + \text{Resource Accessibility} + \text{Virtual Connection} \tag{4.19}$$

**Community Engagement** ($CE$):  Active engagement within online communities is fundamental for digital support.

$$CE = \frac{\text{Participation Level} + \text{Contribution Frequency}}{\text{Community Involvement}} \tag{4.20}$$

**Resource Accessibility** ($RA$):  Accessing diverse resources enhances the support available online.

$$RA = \frac{\text{Information Availability} + \text{Resource Variety}}{\text{Accessibility Rating}} \tag{4.21}$$

**Virtual Connection** ($VC$): Establishing meaningful connections in virtual spaces contributes to the overall online support.

$$VC = \frac{\text{Digital Bonding} + \text{Network Expansion}}{\text{Connection Strength}} \tag{4.22}$$

The combined effect of these online communities and resources components forms the basis for a strong and accessible digital support system:

$$\text{Total Support} = CE + RA + VC \tag{4.23}$$

Additionally, let's represent the concept of digital synergy:

$$\text{Digital Synergy} = \text{Community Engagement} \times \text{Resource Accessibility} \times \text{Virtual Connection} \tag{4.24}$$

This formula underscores the synergistic nature of community engagement, resource accessibility, and virtual connection in building a robust online support system.

Understanding these equations provides individuals with practical tools to harness the power of online communities and resources for a comprehensive support network.

## 4.5  Supportive Networks

Establishing and nurturing supportive networks involves practical insights expressed through mathematical formulas. Let's explore:

$$\text{Network Support Index} = \text{Connection Strength} + \text{Diverse Perspectives} + \text{Reciprocal Assistance} \tag{4.25}$$

**Connection Strength** $(CS)$**:** Fostering strong connections within supportive networks is fundamental.

$$CS = \frac{\text{Interpersonal Bonds} + \text{Communication Resilience}}{\text{Connection Intensity}} \tag{4.26}$$

**Diverse Perspectives** $(DP)$**:** Embracing diverse perspectives enriches the support within networks.

$$DP = \frac{\text{Cultural Diversity} + \text{Varied Experiences}}{\text{Perspective Enrichment}} \tag{4.27}$$

**Reciprocal Assistance** $(RA)$**:** Establishing reciprocal assistance enhances the overall support in networks.

$$RA = \frac{\text{Mutual Aid} + \text{Shared Responsibilities}}{\text{Reciprocal Trust}} \tag{4.28}$$

The combined effect of these supportive network components forms the basis for a strong and reciprocal support system:

$$\text{Total Support} = CS + DP + RA \tag{4.29}$$

Additionally, let's represent the concept of network synergy:

$$\text{Network Synergy} = \text{Connection Strength} \times \text{Diverse Perspectives} \times \text{Reciprocal Assistance} \tag{4.30}$$

This formula underscores the synergistic nature of connection strength, diverse perspectives, and reciprocal assistance in building a robust and supportive network.

Understanding these equations provides individuals with practical tools to cultivate and strengthen their supportive networks for comprehensive and reciprocal support.

## 4.6   Nurturing Relationships

Nurturing and sustaining relationships for support involves practical insights expressed through mathematical formulas. Let's explore:

$$\begin{aligned} \text{Relationship Support Index} = {}& \text{Communication Harmony} + \text{Emotional Resonance} \\ & + \text{Reciprocal Investment} \end{aligned} \tag{4.31}$$

**Communication Harmony** ($CH$): Fostering harmonious communication is fundamental for relationship support.

$$CH = \frac{\text{Effective Communication} + \text{Active Listening}}{\text{Communication Synchronization}} \tag{4.32}$$

**Emotional Resonance** ($ER$): Building emotional resonance contributes to overall support within relationships.

$$ER = \frac{\text{Empathy} + \text{Emotional Connection}}{\text{Emotional Harmony}} \tag{4.33}$$

**Reciprocal Investment** ($RI$): Investing reciprocally in the relationship enhances the overall support.

$$RI = \frac{\text{Shared Efforts} + \text{Mutual Growth}}{\text{Reciprocal Commitment}} \tag{4.34}$$

The combined effect of these nurturing relationship components forms the basis for a strong and reciprocal support system:

$$\text{Total Support} = CH + ER + RI \tag{4.35}$$

Additionally, let's represent the concept of relationship synergy:

$$\text{Relationship Synergy} = \text{Communication Harmony} \times \text{Emotional Resonance} \times \text{Reciprocal Investment} \tag{4.36}$$

This formula underscores the synergistic nature of communication harmony, emotional resonance, and reciprocal investment in building a robust and supportive relationship.

Understanding these equations provides individuals with practical tools to nurture and strengthen their relationships for comprehensive and reciprocal support.

## 4.7   Empathy and Understanding

Cultivating empathy and understanding for support involves practical insights expressed through mathematical formulas. Let's explore:

$$\begin{aligned}\text{Empathy Support Index} = {}& \text{Compassionate Connection} \\ & + \text{Understanding Depth} + \text{Reciprocal Compassion}\end{aligned} \tag{4.37}$$

**Compassionate Connection** ($CC$): Fostering a compassionate connection is fundamental for empathy support.

$$CC = \frac{\text{Sympathetic Bonding} + \text{Active Listening}}{\text{Connection Compassion}} \tag{4.38}$$

**Understanding Depth** ($UD$): Delving into deep understanding contributes to overall support through empathy.

$$UD = \frac{\text{Empathetic Insight} + \text{Perspective Acknowledgment}}{\text{Understanding Intensity}} \tag{4.39}$$

**Reciprocal Compassion** ($RC$): Experiencing reciprocal compassion enhances the overall support.

$$RC = \frac{\text{Shared Empathy} + \text{Mutual Understanding}}{\text{Reciprocal Sympathy}} \tag{4.40}$$

The combined effect of these empathy and understanding components forms the basis for a strong and reciprocal support system:

$$\text{Total Support} = CC + UD + RC \tag{4.41}$$

Additionally, let's represent the concept of empathetic synergy:

$$\text{Empathetic Synergy} = \text{Compassionate Connection} \times \text{Understanding Depth} \times \text{Reciprocal Compassion} \tag{4.42}$$

This formula underscores the synergistic nature of compassionate connection, understanding depth, and reciprocal compassion in building a robust and supportive empathetic environment.

Understanding these equations provides individuals with practical tools to cultivate and strengthen empathy and understanding for comprehensive and reciprocal support.

# Chapter 5

# Mindfulness and Meditation

## 5.1 Introduction to Mindfulness

Introducing mindfulness is essential for mental well-being. Let's explore it through practical insights:

**Mindfulness Equation:**

$$\text{Mindfulness} = \text{Present Moment Awareness} + \text{Non-Judgmental Observation}$$

Mindfulness involves being fully present in the moment and observing without judgment. The equation captures its essence.

**Mindful Breathing Formula:**

$$\text{Mindful Breathing} = \text{Inhalation Time} - \text{Exhalation Time}$$

Practicing mindful breathing, where inhalation and exhalation times are balanced, enhances relaxation and focus.

**Mindfulness in Daily Life:**

$$\text{Daily Mindfulness} = \text{Conscious Eating} + \text{Active Listening} + \text{Purposeful Movements}$$

Incorporating mindfulness into daily activities, like conscious eating and active listening, fosters a mindful lifestyle.

**Mindfulness Benefits:**

$$\text{Mindfulness Benefits} = \text{Stress Reduction} + \text{Improved Focus} + \text{Emotional Regulation}$$

Embracing mindfulness yields numerous benefits, including stress reduction, improved focus, and enhanced emotional regulation.

**Mindfulness Reminder:**

$$\text{Mindfulness Reminder} = \text{Triggered Awareness} + \text{Gentle Redirect}$$

Using a mindfulness reminder involves triggered awareness and gently redirecting attention, reinforcing mindfulness.

Understanding these practical aspects empowers individuals to integrate mindfulness seamlessly into their lives for improved mental well-being.

## 5.2    Meditation Techniques

Exploring practical meditation techniques for a calm mind:

**Breath Awareness:**

$$\text{Breath Awareness} = \text{Conscious Inhalation} + \text{Gentle Exhalation}$$

Focus on conscious breathing, inhaling and exhaling gently, to anchor the mind in the present moment.

**Body Scan Meditation:**

$$\text{Body Scan} = \text{Progressive Relaxation} + \text{Mindful Scanning}$$

Systematically relax each part of the body, combining progressive relaxation with mindful scanning for deep relaxation.

**Loving-Kindness Meditation:**

$$\text{Loving-Kindness} = \text{Self-Compassion} + \text{Universal Well-Wishing}$$

Cultivate a sense of self-compassion and extend well-wishes to others, fostering feelings of love and kindness.

**Mantra Meditation:**

$$\text{Mantra Meditation} = \text{Repetition} + \text{Focused Intention}$$

Repeat a chosen mantra with focused intention, creating a rhythmic and calming meditation practice.

**Visualization Meditation:**

$$\text{Visualization} = \text{Creative Imagery} + \text{Positive Affirmations}$$

Immerse yourself in creative imagery and positive affirmations during meditation for mental clarity and optimism.

**Walking Meditation:**

$$\text{Walking Meditation} = \text{Conscious Steps} + \text{Mindful Breath}$$

Combine conscious walking with mindful breathing, integrating meditation into the act of walking.

**Nature Meditation:**

$$\text{Nature Meditation} = \text{Observation} + \text{Connection}$$

Engage in mindful observation of nature, fostering a deep connection with the natural environment.

**Gratitude Meditation:**

$$\text{Gratitude} = \text{Reflection} + \text{Expressive Thanks}$$

Reflect on gratitude and express thanks during meditation, promoting a positive and grateful mindset.

Incorporating these practical meditation techniques offers diverse ways to cultivate a calm and focused mind.

## 5.3 Mindfulness in Daily Life

Incorporating mindfulness into daily activities for a balanced and mindful lifestyle:

**Mindful Eating Formula:**

$$\text{Mindful Eating} = \text{Conscious Bites} + \text{Savoring Flavors}$$

Savor each bite consciously, engaging all senses, to foster a mindful approach to eating.

**Mindful Communication:**

$$\text{Mindful Communication} = \text{Present Listening} + \text{Thoughtful Response}$$

Listen actively and respond thoughtfully, enhancing communication with a mindful presence.

**Mindful Walking Equation:**

$$\text{Mindful Walking} = \text{Conscious Steps} + \text{Awareness of Movement}$$

Walk with conscious steps, being aware of the movement and connection with the surroundings.

**Mindful Work Productivity:**

$$\text{Mindful Productivity} = \text{Focused Task} + \text{Purposeful Breaks}$$

Approach tasks with focused attention, interspersed with purposeful breaks for enhanced productivity.

**Mindful Technology Use:**

$$\text{Mindful Technology} = \text{Conscious Interaction} + \text{Digital Detox}$$

Interact consciously with technology, balancing it with periodic digital detox for mindful screen time.

**Mindful Driving Technique:**

$$\text{Mindful Driving} = \text{Attentive Observation} + \text{Calm Breath}$$

Drive attentively, incorporating calm breathing techniques for a mindful and safe commute.

**Mindful Time Management:**

$$\text{Mindful Time Management} = \text{Prioritization} + \text{Present Focus}$$

Prioritize tasks mindfully, staying focused on the present to manage time effectively.

**Mindful Relaxation:**

$$\text{Mindful Relaxation} = \text{Conscious Unwinding} + \text{Deep Breathing}$$

Unwind consciously, combining relaxation with deep breathing for a mindful and restful experience.

Practicing mindfulness in daily life involves incorporating these equations into various activities, fostering a balanced and aware lifestyle.

## 5.4 Mindful Breathing Exercises

Engage in practical and easy-to-remember mindful breathing exercises for relaxation and focus:

**Equal Breathing:**

$$\text{Equal Breathing} = \text{Inhalation Time} = \text{Exhalation Time}$$

Inhale and exhale for the same duration, promoting balance and calming the nervous system.

**Box Breathing:**

$$\text{Box Breathing} = \text{Inhale} + \text{Hold} + \text{Exhale} + \text{Hold}$$

Inhale for a count, hold, exhale for the same count, and hold again, forming a box pattern for relaxation.

**4-7-8 Technique:**

$$\text{4-7-8 Technique} = \text{Inhale for } 4 + \text{Hold for } 7 + \text{Exhale for } 8$$

Inhale quietly through the nose for 4 counts, hold the breath for 7 counts, and exhale audibly through the mouth for 8 counts, inducing calmness.

**Alternate Nostril Breathing:**

$$\text{Alternate Nostril Breathing} = \text{Inhale Right} + \text{Exhale Left}$$

Close one nostril, inhale through the other, then close that nostril and exhale through the opposite side, promoting balance.

**Belly Breathing:**

$$\text{Belly Breathing} = \text{Diaphragmatic Expansion} + \text{Relaxed Exhalation}$$

Expand the diaphragm during inhalation, allowing the belly to rise, and exhale slowly for relaxation.

**Ocean Breathing:**

$$\text{Ocean Breathing} = \text{Ujjayi Breath} + \text{Wave-Like Sound}$$

Engage in Ujjayi breath, creating a wave-like sound by constricting the back of the throat for focus and tranquility.

**Mindful Counting:**

$$\text{Mindful Counting} = \text{Conscious Counting} + \text{Gentle Breath Observation}$$

Count each inhalation and exhalation, staying aware and observant of the breath for mindfulness. Incorporating these mindful breathing exercises into your routine provides quick and effective tools for relaxation and concentration.

## 5.5 Cultivating Present-Moment Awareness

Explore practical techniques for cultivating present-moment awareness effortlessly:

**Sensory Grounding:**

$$\text{Sensory Grounding} = \text{Observation of Senses} + \text{Anchor Point Awareness}$$

Engage in mindful observation of the senses, anchoring awareness in a specific point for grounding.

**Mindful Observation:**

$$\text{Mindful Observation} = \text{Focused Attention} + \text{Non-Judgmental Awareness}$$

Observe surroundings with focused attention, maintaining non-judgmental awareness for present-moment connection.

**Five Senses Check-In:**

$$\text{Five Senses Check-In} = \text{Sight} + \text{Sound} + \text{Touch} + \text{Taste} + \text{Smell}$$

Conduct a quick check-in of the five senses, connecting with each one for heightened present-moment awareness.

**Breath as Anchor:**

$$\text{Breath as Anchor} = \text{Conscious Breathing} + \text{Centering Breath Awareness}$$

Use conscious breathing as an anchor, centering awareness on the breath for immediate present-moment connection.

**Body Scan Awareness:**

$$\text{Body Scan Awareness} = \text{Gradual Scan} + \text{Tension Release}$$

Systematically scan the body, releasing tension and fostering present-moment awareness.

**Nature Connection:**

$$\text{Nature Connection} = \text{Outdoor Presence} + \text{Environmental Sensing}$$

Connect with nature, sensing the outdoor environment to enhance present-moment awareness.

**Mindful Reflection:**

$$\text{Mindful Reflection} = \text{Thought Observation} + \text{Detached Reflection}$$

Observe thoughts without attachment, reflecting mindfully on the present moment.

Incorporating these techniques effortlessly into daily life promotes a natural and continuous cultivation of present-moment awareness.

## 5.6   Mindful Decision-Making

Explore practical techniques for making mindful decisions with ease:

**Decision Clarity Formula:**

$$\text{Decision Clarity} = \text{Reflective Contemplation} + \text{Objective Evaluation}$$

Contemplate decisions reflectively and evaluate them objectively for clarity.

**Mindful Prioritization:**

$$\text{Mindful Prioritization} = \text{Value Alignment} + \text{Intentional Focus}$$

Align decisions with personal values and maintain intentional focus for mindful prioritization.

**Emotional Regulation in Decision-Making:**

$$\text{Emotional Regulation} = \text{Breath Awareness} + \text{Emotion Acknowledgment}$$

Utilize breath awareness and acknowledge emotions for effective emotional regulation in decision-making.

**Pros and Cons Balance:**

$$\text{Pros and Cons Balance} = \text{Positive Aspects} - \text{Negative Aspects}$$

Evaluate the positive and negative aspects of decisions, seeking balance for informed choices.

**Intuitive Decision-Making:**

$$\text{Intuitive Decision-Making} = \text{Gut Feeling} + \text{Instinct Recognition}$$

Trust gut feelings and recognize instincts as valuable inputs in decision-making.

**Mindful Commitment:**

$$\text{Mindful Commitment} = \text{Clear Intent} + \text{Conscious Action}$$

Commit to decisions with clear intent and engage in conscious actions for mindful commitment.

**Decision Reflection:**

$$\text{Decision Reflection} = \text{Outcome Evaluation} + \text{Lesson Integration}$$

Reflect on decision outcomes, integrating lessons learned for continuous improvement.

Incorporating these practical techniques into decision-making processes ensures a mindful and balanced approach to choices.

## 5.7   Mindfulness for Stress Reduction

Explore practical techniques for utilizing mindfulness to reduce stress effortlessly:

**Stress Awareness Equation:**

$$\text{Stress Awareness} = \text{Conscious Recognition} + \text{Emotion Acknowledgment}$$

Be consciously aware of stress, acknowledging emotions associated with it for proactive management.

**Mindful Breathing for Stress Relief:**

$$\text{Mindful Breathing for Stress Relief} = \text{Inhalation Time} - \text{Exhalation Time}$$

Engage in mindful breathing, where inhalation and exhalation times are balanced, for immediate stress relief.

**Mindful Body Scan:**

$$\text{Mindful Body Scan} = \text{Tension Identification} + \text{Progressive Relaxation}$$

Identify tension in the body and systematically relax each part through mindful body scanning.

**Present Moment Anchoring:**

$$\text{Present Moment Anchoring} = \text{Anchor Point Focus} + \text{Observation Clarity}$$

Focus on an anchor point in the present moment, enhancing observation clarity for stress reduction.

**Mindful Reflection on Stressors:**

$$\text{Mindful Reflection on Stressors} = \text{Stressor Identification} + \text{Detached Reflection}$$

Identify stressors and reflect on them without attachment, fostering a mindful approach to stress.

**Cognitive Restructuring:**

$$\text{Cognitive Restructuring} = \text{Thought Reframing} + \text{Positive Affirmation Integration}$$

Reframe negative thoughts and integrate positive affirmations for a more resilient mindset.

**Mindful Gratitude Practice:**

$$\text{Mindful Gratitude Practice} = \text{Gratitude Reflection} + \text{Expressive Thanks}$$

Reflect on moments of gratitude and express thanks, cultivating a positive mindset amidst stress.

Incorporating these practical mindfulness techniques into daily life provides effective tools for reducing stress and promoting overall well-being.

# Chapter 6

# Cognitive Behavioral Therapy (CBT)

## 6.1 Principles of CBT

Explore the foundational principles of Cognitive Behavioral Therapy (CBT) in a practical and memorable manner:

**Thought-Behavior Connection:**

$$\text{Thought-Behavior Connection} = \text{Awareness of Thoughts} + \text{Behavioral Response}$$

Be aware of thoughts and recognize their impact on behavior, fostering conscious and intentional responses.

**Cognitive Restructuring Equation:**

$$\text{Cognitive Restructuring} = \text{Identifying Negative Thoughts} + \text{Positive Thought Integration}$$

Identify negative thoughts and replace them with positive alternatives through cognitive restructuring.

**Behavioral Activation Formula:**

$$\text{Behavioral Activation} = \text{Activity Planning} + \text{Goal-Oriented Behavior}$$

Engage in planned activities and set goal-oriented behaviors to enhance mood and motivation.

**Exposure Therapy Approach:**

$$\text{Exposure Therapy Approach} = \text{Gradual Exposure} + \text{Fear Reduction}$$

Gradually expose oneself to feared situations, reducing anxiety and enhancing adaptive responses.

**Mindfulness Integration:**

$$\text{Mindfulness Integration} = \text{Present-Moment Awareness} + \text{Non-Judgmental Observation}$$

Incorporate mindfulness techniques for present-moment awareness and non-judgmental observation.

**Problem-Solving Equation:**

$$\text{Problem-Solving} = \text{Problem Identification} + \text{Solution Development}$$

Identify problems and develop practical solutions through systematic problem-solving.

**CBT ABC Model:**

$$\text{CBT ABC Model} = \text{Activating Event} + \text{Beliefs about Event} + \text{Consequence of Beliefs}$$

Analyze events through the ABC model: Activating Event, Beliefs about Event, and Consequence of Beliefs.

Incorporating these principles empowers individuals to apply CBT techniques for effective self-help and personal growth.

## 6.2    Identifying and Changing Negative Thoughts

Discover practical techniques for identifying and changing negative thoughts effortlessly:

**Negative Thought Recognition:**

$$\text{Negative Thought Recognition} = \text{Thought Awareness} + \text{Emotion Connection}$$

Be aware of negative thoughts and connect them to associated emotions for effective recognition.

**Cognitive Restructuring Formula:**

$$\text{Cognitive Restructuring} = \text{Challenging Negative Thoughts} + \text{Positive Thought Integration}$$

Challenge negative thoughts and integrate positive alternatives through cognitive restructuring.

**Automatic Thought Analysis:**

$$\text{Automatic Thought Analysis} = \text{Identification} + \text{Rational Examination}$$

Identify automatic negative thoughts and subject them to rational examination for perspective.

**Socratic Questioning for Thoughts:**

$$\text{Socratic Questioning} = \text{Exploration of Assumptions} + \text{Alternative Perspectives}$$

Explore assumptions behind thoughts and consider alternative perspectives using Socratic questioning.

**Behavioral Experiments for Thoughts:**

$$\text{Behavioral Experiments} = \text{Testing Assumptions} + \text{Observing Outcomes}$$

Test assumptions through behavioral experiments and observe outcomes for practical insight.

**Mindfulness Integration:**

$$\text{Mindfulness Integration} = \text{Present Moment Observation} + \text{Non-Judgmental Awareness}$$

Integrate mindfulness into thought processes by observing the present moment with non-judgmental awareness.

**Positive Affirmation Adoption:**

$$\text{Positive Affirmation Adoption} = \text{Affirmation Selection} + \text{Daily Integration}$$

Select positive affirmations and integrate them daily to counteract negative thoughts.

Incorporating these practical CBT techniques empowers individuals to identify and change negative thoughts effectively for improved mental well-being.

## 6.3 Behavioral Activation

Explore practical techniques for Behavioral Activation, promoting positive behaviors and mood improvement:

**Activity Planning Formula:**

$$\text{Activity Planning} = \text{Goal Setting} + \text{Task Breakdown}$$

Set realistic goals and break them down into manageable tasks for effective activity planning.

**Behavioral Experimentation:**

$$Behavioral\ Experimentation = New\ Activity\ Introduction + Outcome\ Observation$$

Introduce new activities and observe outcomes through behavioral experimentation for positive reinforcement.

**Reward System Integration:**

$$Reward\ System\ Integration = Activity\ Reward\ Identification + Reinforcement\ Application$$

Identify rewards associated with activities and apply reinforcement to enhance motivation.

**Routine Development Equation:**

$$Routine\ Development = Consistent\ Activity\ Scheduling + Adaptation\ for\ Variety$$

Schedule activities consistently and adapt routines to include a variety of positive behaviors.

**Social Engagement Strategy:**

$$Social\ Engagement = Connection\ Initiatives + Quality\ Interaction$$

Initiate social connections and focus on the quality of interactions for behavioral activation.

**Graded Exposure Technique:**

$$Graded\ Exposure = Stepwise\ Challenge + Anxiety\ Monitoring$$

Gradually expose oneself to challenges, monitoring anxiety levels for effective behavioral activation.

**Mindful Activity Participation:**

$$Mindful\ Activity\ Participation = Present\ Moment\ Engagement + Mindful\ Reflection$$

Engage in activities mindfully, being present in the moment, and reflect on the experience.

Incorporating these practical Behavioral Activation techniques fosters positive behaviors and contributes to overall mood improvement in the context of Cognitive Behavioral Therapy.

## 6.4   CBT for Anxiety and Depression

Explore practical techniques for applying CBT to manage anxiety and depression effortlessly:

**Thought Restructuring for Anxiety:**

Thought Restructuring for Anxiety = Identify Anxious Thoughts + Challenge Irrational Beliefs

Identify anxious thoughts and challenge irrational beliefs through thought restructuring.

**Behavioral Activation for Depression:**

Behavioral Activation for Depression = Gradual Activity Introduction + Positive Reinforcement

Gradually introduce activities and incorporate positive reinforcement to alleviate symptoms of depression.

**Exposure Therapy for Anxiety:**

Exposure Therapy for Anxiety = Gradual Exposure + Anxiety Habituation

Gradually expose oneself to anxiety triggers, promoting habituation for reduced anxiety response.

**Mindfulness-Based CBT Techniques:**

Mindfulness-Based CBT Techniques = Present Moment Awareness + Cognitive Reframing

Incorporate mindfulness practices with cognitive reframing to enhance coping with anxiety and depression.

**Problem-Solving for Depression:**

Problem-Solving for Depression = Identify Problem Areas + Generate Solutions

Identify problem areas contributing to depression and generate practical solutions through problem-solving.

**Relaxation Techniques for Anxiety:**

Relaxation Techniques for Anxiety = Deep Breathing + Progressive Muscle Relaxation

Utilize deep breathing and progressive muscle relaxation for immediate relief from anxiety symptoms.

**Positive Self-Talk Integration:**

Positive Self-Talk Integration = Affirmation Adoption + Challenge Negative Self-Talk

Adopt positive affirmations and challenge negative self-talk for a more positive mindset.

Incorporating these practical CBT techniques provides effective tools for managing anxiety and depression, fostering mental well-being.

# 6.5   Cognitive Restructuring

Discover practical techniques for Cognitive Restructuring, reshaping thought patterns effortlessly:

**Automatic Thought Analysis:**

$$\text{Automatic Thought Analysis} = \text{Identification} + \text{Rational Examination}$$

Identify automatic negative thoughts and subject them to rational examination for perspective.

**Cognitive Reframing Formula:**

$$\text{Cognitive Reframing} = \text{Positive Perspective Integration} + \text{Challenge Negative Beliefs}$$

Integrate positive perspectives and challenge negative beliefs through cognitive reframing.

**Socratic Questioning for Thoughts:**

$$\text{Socratic Questioning} = \text{Exploration of Assumptions} + \text{Alternative Perspectives}$$

Explore assumptions behind thoughts and consider alternative perspectives using Socratic questioning.

**Mindful Thought Observation:**

$$\text{Mindful Thought Observation} = \text{Present Moment Awareness} + \text{Non-Judgmental Observation}$$

Observe thoughts mindfully in the present moment, practicing non-judgmental awareness.

**Behavioral Experiments for Thoughts:**

$$\text{Behavioral Experiments} = \text{Testing Assumptions} + \text{Observing Outcomes}$$

Test assumptions through behavioral experiments and observe outcomes for practical insight.

**Positive Affirmation Integration:**

$$\text{Positive Affirmation Integration} = \text{Affirmation Selection} + \text{Daily Integration}$$

Select positive affirmations and integrate them daily to counteract negative thoughts.

**Thought Journaling for Awareness:**

$$\text{Thought Journaling for Awareness} = \text{Record Thoughts} + \text{Emotion Reflection}$$

Record thoughts in a journal and reflect on associated emotions for heightened self-awareness.

Incorporating these practical Cognitive Restructuring techniques empowers individuals to reshape thought patterns and promote positive mental well-being.

# 6.6 Building Healthy Habits

Discover practical techniques for building and sustaining healthy habits effortlessly:

**Habit Formation Equation:**

$$\text{Habit Formation} = \text{Cue Recognition} + \text{Routine Establishment} + \text{Reward Integration}$$

Recognize cues, establish routines, and integrate rewards for effective habit formation.

**SMART Goal Setting:**

$$\text{SMART Goal Setting} = \text{Specificity} + \text{Measurability} + \text{Achievability} + \text{Relevance} + \text{Time-bound}$$

Set Specific, Measurable, Achievable, Relevant, and Time-bound goals for successful habit building.

**Behavioral Activation for Habits:**

$$\text{Behavioral Activation for Habits} = \text{Task Breakdown} + \text{Positive Reinforcement}$$

Break down tasks and apply positive reinforcement to activate and maintain healthy habits.

**Habit Loop Modification:**

$$\text{Habit Loop Modification} = \text{Cue Replacement} + \text{Behavioral Substitution} + \text{Reward Adjustment}$$

Modify the habit loop by replacing cues, substituting behaviors, and adjusting rewards.

**Implementation Intentions:**

$$\text{Implementation Intentions} = \text{Anticipate Challenges} + \text{Plan Responses}$$

Anticipate challenges and plan specific responses to overcome obstacles in habit formation.

**Tracking Progress Formula:**

$$\text{Tracking Progress} = \text{Regular Evaluation} + \text{Adjustment for Improvement}$$

Regularly evaluate progress and adjust habits for continuous improvement.

**Mindful Habit Integration:**

$$\text{Mindful Habit Integration} = \text{Present Moment Engagement} + \text{Non-Judgmental Reflection}$$

Integrate habits mindfully, engaging in the present moment with non-judgmental reflection.

Incorporating these practical techniques into daily life empowers individuals to build and sustain healthy habits, contributing to overall well-being.

## 6.7   CBT Tools for Everyday Challenges

Explore practical CBT tools for navigating everyday challenges effortlessly:

**ABC Model for Challenging Situations:**

$$ABC\ Model = Activating\ Event\ Identification + Belief\ Examination + Consequence\ Evaluation$$

Identify activating events, examine beliefs associated with them, and evaluate consequences for a rational response.

**Coping Cards for Stress Management:**

$$Coping\ Cards = Positive\ Coping\ Strategies + Immediate\ Application$$

Compile coping cards with positive strategies for immediate application in stressful situations.

**Thought Record Sheet for Perspective Shift:**

$$Thought\ Record\ Sheet = Record\ Automatic\ Thoughts + Challenge\ and\ Reframe$$

Record automatic thoughts, challenge them, and reframe for a more balanced perspective.

**Behavioral Experimentation for Decision-Making:**

$$Behavioral\ Experimentation = Decision\ Identification + Testing\ Assumptions$$

Identify decisions, test assumptions through behavioral experiments for informed choices.

**Gratitude Journal for Positive Outlook:**

$$Gratitude\ Journal = Daily\ Gratitude\ Reflection + Positive\ Affirmation\ Integration$$

Reflect on daily gratitude and integrate positive affirmations for a positive outlook.

**Five-Column Technique for Problem-Solving:**

$$Five\text{-}Column\ Technique = Problem\ Identification + Generate\ Solutions + Choose\ Action$$

Identify problems, generate solutions, and choose actionable steps for effective problem-solving.

**Visualization for Goal Achievement:**

$$Visualization = Imagining\ Success + Emotional\ Connection$$

Visualize success and emotionally connect with the desired outcome for motivation.

Incorporating these practical CBT tools into daily life equips individuals with effective strategies for navigating everyday challenges and promoting mental resilience.

# Chapter 7

# Medication and Psychiatry

## 7.1  Overview of Psychiatric Medications

Explore a quick and practical overview of psychiatric medications:

**Antidepressants:** Antidepressants, like SSRIs (Selective Serotonin Reuptake Inhibitors) and SNRIs (Serotonin-Norepinephrine Reuptake Inhibitors), enhance serotonin levels in the brain, improving mood and alleviating depression.

**Anxiolytics:** Anxiolytics, such as benzodiazepines, act on the central nervous system to reduce anxiety and promote relaxation.

**Antipsychotics:** Antipsychotics, including typical and atypical variants, manage symptoms of psychosis, such as hallucinations and delusions.

**Mood Stabilizers:** Mood stabilizers, like lithium, help regulate mood and prevent extreme shifts in emotions, commonly used in bipolar disorder treatment.

**Stimulants:** Stimulants, such as methylphenidate or amphetamines, enhance neurotransmitter activity, often prescribed for attention-deficit/hyperactivity disorder (ADHD).

**Anticonvulsants:** Anticonvulsants, like valproate, have mood-stabilizing effects and are used to treat conditions like bipolar disorder.

**Beta Blockers:** Beta blockers, such as propranolol, may be used to alleviate physical symptoms of anxiety, like rapid heartbeat.

**Sleep Aids:** Sleep aids, including hypnotic medications, help regulate sleep patterns and treat insomnia.

**Calculation for Medication Dosage:**

$$\text{Medication Dosage} = \text{Patient Weight} \times \text{Dosage per kg}$$

Calculate medication dosage based on patient weight and recommended dosage per kilogram.

**Chemical Formula for a Common Antidepressant (e.g., Sertraline):**

$$C_{17}H_{17}Cl_2N$$

Presenting the chemical formula of a common antidepressant for reference.

Incorporating these insights into psychiatric medications provides a practical understanding of their functions and applications.

## 7.2  Working with Mental Health Professionals

Explore practical tips for collaborating with mental health professionals:

**Communication Equation:**

$$\text{Effective Communication} = \text{Active Listening} + \text{Expressing Concerns} + \text{Clarifying Information}$$

Foster effective communication by actively listening, expressing concerns, and clarifying information during sessions.

**Appointment Scheduling Formula:**

$$\text{Appointment Scheduling} = \text{Frequency of Sessions} + \text{Consistency}$$

Establish a consistent schedule for therapy sessions to ensure regular and meaningful engagement.

**Goal-Setting Techniques:**

$$\text{Goal-Setting} = \text{Collaborative Goal Identification} + \text{SMART Goals}$$

Identify collaborative goals with your mental health professional and set Specific, Measurable, Achievable, Relevant, and Time-bound objectives.

**Medication Adherence Strategies:**

$$\text{Medication Adherence} = \text{Daily Routine Integration} + \text{Reminder Systems}$$

Integrate medications into daily routines and use reminder systems to enhance adherence.

**Emergency Contact Plan:**

$$\text{Emergency Contact Plan} = \text{Identifying Emergency Contacts} + \text{Crisis Response Plan}$$

Develop an emergency contact plan, including crisis response strategies, for unexpected situations.

**Therapeutic Techniques Utilization:**

$$\text{Therapeutic Techniques} = \text{Homework Completion} + \text{Application in Daily Life}$$

Maximize therapeutic benefits by completing assigned homework and applying learned techniques in daily life.

**Feedback Integration:**

$$\text{Feedback Integration} = \text{Constructive Feedback Reception} + \text{Open Communication}$$

Receive constructive feedback openly and maintain open communication with your mental health professional.

**Chemical Equation for a Stress-Reducing Neurotransmitter (e.g., Serotonin):**

$$C_{10}H_{12}N_2O$$

Presenting the chemical formula of a stress-reducing neurotransmitter for reference.

Incorporating these practical tips enhances collaboration with mental health professionals, fostering a supportive and effective therapeutic relationship.

## 7.3 Managing Medication Side Effects

Explore practical tips for managing medication side effects:

**Hydration Formula:**

$$\text{Hydration} = \text{Daily Water Intake} + \text{Monitoring Hydration Levels}$$

Maintain proper hydration by monitoring daily water intake and hydration levels, especially for medications affecting fluid balance.

**Nutritional Support Equation:**

$$\text{Nutritional Support} = \text{Balanced Diet} + \text{Supplement Consideration}$$

Support overall health with a balanced diet and consider supplements to address nutritional deficiencies caused by medication.

**Sleep Hygiene Techniques:**

$$\text{Sleep Hygiene} = \text{Consistent Sleep Schedule} + \text{Sleep Environment Optimization}$$

Improve sleep quality by maintaining a consistent sleep schedule and optimizing the sleep environment, crucial for medications influencing sleep.

**Physical Activity Integration:**

$$\text{Physical Activity} = \text{Daily Exercise} + \text{Adaptation to Medication Effects}$$

Incorporate daily exercise and adapt physical activity routines to mitigate medication-related effects on energy levels.

**Cognitive Strategies for Cognitive Side Effects:**

$$\text{Cognitive Strategies} = \text{Memory Exercises} + \text{Mental Stimulation Activities}$$

Counter cognitive side effects with memory exercises and engaging mental stimulation activities.

**Monitoring Vital Signs:**

$$\text{Vital Signs Monitoring} = \text{Blood Pressure Checks} + \text{Heart Rate Evaluation}$$

Regularly monitor vital signs, including blood pressure and heart rate, for medications affecting cardiovascular health.

**Chemical Formula for a Common Antipsychotic Medication (e.g., Olanzapine):**

$$C_{17}H_{20}N_4S$$

Presenting the chemical formula of a common antipsychotic medication for reference.

**Collaborative Communication with Healthcare Provider:**

$$\text{Collaborative Communication} = \text{Reporting Side Effects} + \text{Adjustment Discussions}$$

Maintain collaborative communication with healthcare providers by promptly reporting side effects and engaging in discussions about medication adjustments.

Incorporating these practical tips empowers individuals to manage medication side effects effectively, optimizing overall well-being.

## 7.4   Finding the Right Medication

Explore practical tips for finding the right medication:

**Symptom Tracking System:**

$$\text{Symptom Tracking} = \text{Daily Symptom Journal} + \text{Severity Rating}$$

Establish a symptom tracking system using a daily journal and severity rating to identify patterns and assess medication effectiveness.

**Open Communication with Healthcare Provider:**

$$\text{Open Communication} = \text{Expressing Concerns} + \text{Reporting Changes}$$

Maintain open communication with healthcare providers by expressing concerns and promptly reporting any changes in symptoms.

**Genetic Testing Consideration:**

$$\text{Genetic Testing} = \text{Pharmacogenomic Analysis} + \text{Medication Response Prediction}$$

Consider genetic testing, such as pharmacogenomic analysis, for predicting individual responses to medications.

**Dose Adjustment Formula:**

$$\text{Dose Adjustment} = \text{Gradual Titration} + \text{Monitoring Side Effects}$$

Facilitate the finding of the right dose by gradually titrating and closely monitoring side effects.

**Medication Rotation Strategy:**

$$\text{Medication Rotation} = \text{Switching Medications} + \text{Monitoring Response}$$

Implement a medication rotation strategy by switching medications and monitoring responses to optimize treatment.

**Feedback Integration System:**

$$\text{Feedback Integration} = \text{Patient Feedback} + \text{Healthcare Provider Evaluation}$$

Integrate patient feedback with healthcare provider evaluations to guide medication adjustments.

**Trial Period Consideration:**

$$\text{Trial Period} = \text{Defined Timeframe} + \text{Regular Evaluation}$$

Establish a defined trial period for medications, conducting regular evaluations to determine effectiveness.

**Chemical Formula for a Common Antianxiety Medication (e.g., Diazepam):**

$$C`16H`13ClN`2O$$

Presenting the chemical formula of a common antianxiety medication for reference.

Incorporating these practical tips streamlines the process of finding the right medication, enhancing the overall treatment experience.

## 7.5   Psychiatric Evaluation

Explore practical aspects of a psychiatric evaluation:

**Self-Assessment Equation:**

$$\text{Self-Assessment} = \text{Reflective Journaling} + \text{Emotional Inventory}$$

Initiate a self-assessment using reflective journaling and an emotional inventory to provide insights during the evaluation.

**Symptom Presentation Techniques:**

$$\text{Symptom Presentation} = \text{Clear Descriptions} + \text{Contextual Examples}$$

Effectively communicate symptoms with clear descriptions and contextual examples to aid the evaluation process.

**Emotional Scale Utilization:**

$$\text{Emotional Scale} = \text{Rating Intensity} + \text{Frequency Assessment}$$

Use an emotional scale to rate the intensity and assess the frequency of emotions experienced.

**Functional Impairment Evaluation:**

$$\text{Functional Impairment} = \text{Daily Functioning Assessment} + \text{Impact on Activities}$$

Evaluate functional impairment by assessing daily functioning and understanding the impact on various activities.

**Personal History Documentation:**

$$\text{Personal History} = \text{Life Events Timeline} + \text{Relevant Experiences}$$

Document personal history through a timeline of life events and highlighting relevant experiences.

**Collaborative Goal Setting Formula:**

$$\text{Collaborative Goal Setting} = \text{Identifying Goals} + \text{Prioritization}$$

Collaborate on goal setting by identifying priorities and establishing a roadmap for treatment.

**Therapeutic Alliance Enhancement:**

$$\text{Therapeutic Alliance} = \text{Open Communication} + \text{Trust Building}$$

Enhance the therapeutic alliance through open communication and actively building trust with the healthcare provider.

**Chemical Formula for a Common Mood Stabilizer (e.g., Lithium):**

$$LiC\cdot 6H\cdot 5O\cdot 7$$

Presenting the chemical formula of a common mood stabilizer for reference.

Incorporating these practical aspects into a psychiatric evaluation fosters a collaborative and insightful approach to mental health assessment.

# 7.6 Collaborative Treatment Plans

Explore practical aspects of collaborative treatment planning:

**Goal Setting Framework:**

$$\text{Goal Setting} = \text{SMART Goals} + \text{Patient Priorities}$$

Establish SMART goals collaboratively, incorporating patient priorities for a personalized treatment plan.

**Medication Adherence Equation:**

$$\text{Medication Adherence} = \text{Daily Routine Integration} + \text{Reminder Systems}$$

Enhance medication adherence by integrating medications into daily routines and utilizing reminder systems.

**Therapeutic Interventions Matrix:**

$$\text{Therapeutic Interventions} = \text{Psychotherapy Options} + \text{Medication Strategies}$$

Create a matrix of therapeutic interventions, combining psychotherapy options and medication strategies for comprehensive treatment.

**Regular Progress Assessment:**

$$\text{Progress Assessment} = \text{Monthly Check-ins} + \text{Adjustment Discussions}$$

Conduct regular progress assessments through monthly check-ins and discussions about potential treatment adjustments.

**Crisis Response Plan Equation:**

$$\text{Crisis Response Plan} = \text{Emergency Contacts} + \text{De-escalation Techniques}$$

Develop a crisis response plan with identified emergency contacts and de-escalation techniques for unexpected situations.

**Collaborative Decision-Making Formula:**

$$\text{Collaborative Decision-Making} = \text{Informed Consent} + \text{Shared Decision-Making}$$

Facilitate collaborative decision-making through informed consent and shared decision-making processes.

**Holistic Wellness Integration:**

$$\text{Holistic Wellness} = \text{Mind-Body Practices} + \text{Lifestyle Adjustments}$$

Integrate holistic wellness into the treatment plan, combining mind-body practices and lifestyle adjustments.

**Chemical Formula for a Common Antidepressant (e.g., Sertraline):**

$$C{\cdot}17H{\cdot}17Cl{\cdot}2N$$

Presenting the chemical formula of a common antidepressant for reference.

Incorporating these practical aspects into collaborative treatment plans ensures a holistic and patient-centered approach to mental health.


## 7.7   Monitoring Medication Efficacy

Explore practical aspects of monitoring medication efficacy:

**Symptom Tracking System:**

$$\text{Symptom Tracking} = \text{Daily Symptom Journal} + \text{Severity Rating}$$

Initiate a symptom tracking system using a daily journal and severity ratings to monitor changes and assess medication efficacy.

**Functional Improvement Index:**

$$\text{Functional Improvement} = \text{Daily Functioning Scale} + \text{Task Accomplishment Rate}$$

Assess functional improvement through a daily functioning scale and task accomplishment rate, measuring the impact of medications on daily activities.

**Emotional Resilience Equation:**

$$\text{Emotional Resilience} = \text{Stress Response Assessment} + \text{Adaptive Coping Strategies}$$

Evaluate emotional resilience by assessing stress response and identifying adaptive coping strategies influenced by medication.

**Quality of Life Measurement:**

$$\text{Quality of Life} = \text{Life Satisfaction Index} + \text{Social Engagement Evaluation}$$

Measure quality of life using a life satisfaction index and evaluating social engagement, considering the broader impact of medication.

**Cognitive Functioning Matrix:**

$$\text{Cognitive Functioning} = \text{Memory Tests} + \text{Concentration Assessment}$$

Monitor cognitive functioning through memory tests and concentration assessments, observing any changes influenced by medication.

**Sleep Quality Index:**

$$\text{Sleep Quality} = \text{Sleep Duration} + \text{Sleep Disturbance Rating}$$

Assess sleep quality by tracking sleep duration and using a sleep disturbance rating, crucial in evaluating medication impact.

**Chemical Formula for a Common Antipsychotic Medication (e.g., Risperidone):**

$$C_{23}H_{27}FN_4O_2$$

Presenting the chemical formula of a common antipsychotic medication for reference.

**Regular Communication Schedule:**

$$\text{Communication Schedule} = \text{Monthly Check-ins} + \text{Adverse Effects Reporting}$$

Establish a regular communication schedule with healthcare providers, including monthly check-ins and reporting any adverse effects promptly.

Incorporating these practical aspects into monitoring medication efficacy ensures a comprehensive and patient-focused approach to mental health care.

# Chapter 8

# Setting and Achieving Goals

## 8.1   SMART Goal Setting

Explore practical aspects of SMART goal setting:

**Specificity Formula:**

$$\text{Specificity} = \text{Clear Objective} + \text{Detailed Actions}$$

Enhance specificity by formulating a clear objective and defining detailed actions required for goal achievement.

**Measurability Equation:**

$$\text{Measurability} = \text{Quantifiable Criteria} + \text{Progress Tracking}$$

Ensure measurability by establishing quantifiable criteria and implementing a system for tracking progress.

**Achievability Matrix:**

$$\text{Achievability} = \text{Skill Assessment} + \text{Resource Availability}$$

Assess achievability by evaluating personal skills and considering the availability of necessary resources.

**Relevance Assessment:**

$$\text{Relevance} = \text{Alignment with Values} + \text{Long-Term Vision}$$

Determine relevance by aligning goals with personal values and considering their contribution to long-term vision.

**Time-Bound Framework:**

$$\text{Time-Bound} = \text{Defined Timeline} + \text{Periodic Checkpoints}$$

Implement a time-bound framework by setting a defined timeline and establishing periodic checkpoints for assessment.

**Goal Attainment Equation:**

$$\text{Goal Attainment} = \text{Regular Review} + \text{Adjustment Strategies}$$

Achieve goals through regular reviews and the implementation of adjustment strategies to address evolving needs.

**Chemical Formula for a Common Motivational Neurotransmitter (e.g., Dopamine):**

$$C_8H_{11}NO_2$$

Presenting the chemical formula of a common motivational neurotransmitter for reference.

**Feedback Integration System:**

$$\text{Feedback Integration} = \text{Self-Reflection} + \text{External Feedback}$$

Integrate feedback into goal setting by incorporating self-reflection and seeking external input for continuous improvement.

Incorporating these practical aspects into SMART goal setting enhances the clarity, effectiveness, and achievability of personal objectives.

## 8.2   Breaking Down Large Goals

Explore practical aspects of breaking down large goals:

**Decomposition Strategy:**

$$\text{Decomposition} = \text{Divide into Smaller Tasks} + \text{Sequential Order}$$

Implement a decomposition strategy by dividing large goals into smaller, manageable tasks with a defined sequential order.

**Task Duration Estimation Formula:**

$$\text{Task Duration} = \text{Time Required per Task} + \text{Buffer for Unexpected Delays}$$

Estimate task duration by considering the time required per task and including a buffer for unexpected delays.

**Resource Allocation Matrix:**

$$\text{Resource Allocation} = \text{Identify Necessary Resources} + \text{Optimal Utilization}$$

Allocate resources effectively by identifying what is necessary for each task and ensuring optimal utilization.

**Priority Scoring System:**

$$\text{Priority Score} = \text{Impact on Overall Goal} + \text{Urgency}$$

Assign priority scores to tasks based on their impact on the overall goal and the level of urgency involved.

**Visual Progress Tracking:**

$$\text{Visual Progress} = \text{Progress Chart} + \text{Completion Milestones}$$

Track progress visually by creating a progress chart and marking completion milestones for motivation.

**Feedback Loop Integration:**

$$\text{Feedback Loop} = \text{Regular Review} + \text{Adaptation Strategies}$$

Integrate a feedback loop by conducting regular reviews and implementing adaptation strategies as needed.

**Chemical Formula for a Common Stress-Reducing Hormone (e.g., Oxytocin):**

$$C\cdot43H\cdot66N\cdot12O\cdot12S\cdot2$$

Presenting the chemical formula of a common stress-reducing hormone for reference.

**Celebration and Reflection Equation:**

$$\text{Celebration and Reflection} = \text{Goal Milestone Celebrations} + \text{Reflect on Lessons Learned}$$

Celebrate goal milestones and reflect on lessons learned, fostering continuous improvement.

Incorporating these practical aspects into breaking down large goals enhances the manageability and success of the overall goal achievement process.

## 8.3 Celebrating Successes

Explore practical aspects of celebrating successes:

**Reward System Integration:**

$$Reward\ System = Define\ Achievable\ Milestones + Meaningful\ Rewards$$

Integrate a reward system by defining achievable milestones and attaching meaningful rewards to celebrate success.

**Recognition Formula:**

$$Recognition = Public\ Acknowledgment + Team\ Celebrations$$

Acknowledge success through public recognition and team celebrations, fostering a positive and motivating environment.

**Reflection and Gratitude Equation:**

$$Reflection\ and\ Gratitude = Reflect\ on\ Achievements + Express\ Gratitude$$

Celebrate successes by reflecting on achievements and expressing gratitude for the contributions of oneself and others.

**Social Connection Index:**

$$Social\ Connection = Celebration\ Events + Sharing\ Success\ Stories$$

Strengthen social connections by organizing celebration events and sharing success stories within the community.

**Self-Appreciation Algorithm:**

$$Self\text{-}Appreciation = Positive\ Self\text{-}Talk + Self\text{-}Rewards$$

Promote self-appreciation through positive self-talk and rewarding oneself for accomplishments, fostering self-esteem.

**Chemical Formula for a Common Happiness Neurotransmitter (e.g., Serotonin):**

$$C_{10}H_{12}N_2O$$

Presenting the chemical formula of a common happiness neurotransmitter for reference.

**Goal Visualization Technique:**

$$\text{Goal Visualization} = \text{Imagining Success Scenes} + \text{Emotional Connection}$$

Enhance goal achievement by visualizing success scenes and establishing an emotional connection to the desired outcomes.

**Continual Improvement Loop:**

$$\text{Continual Improvement} = \text{Feedback Incorporation} + \text{Setting New Challenges}$$

Create a continual improvement loop by incorporating feedback and setting new challenges after celebrating successes.

Incorporating these practical aspects into celebrating successes ensures a positive and motivating atmosphere, encouraging sustained effort and goal pursuit.

## 8.4 Adjusting Goals as Needed

Explore practical aspects of adjusting goals as needed:

**Flexibility Equation:**

$$\text{Flexibility} = \text{Adaptation Strategies} + \text{Openness to Change}$$

Incorporate flexibility by implementing adaptation strategies and maintaining openness to change as needed.

**Feedback Utilization Formula:**

$$\text{Feedback Utilization} = \text{Constructive Feedback Analysis} + \text{Adjustment Implementation}$$

Utilize feedback effectively by analyzing constructive feedback and implementing necessary adjustments to goals.

**Relevance Reassessment System:**

$$\text{Relevance Reassessment} = \text{Current Priorities Evaluation} + \text{Alignment with Values}$$

Reassess relevance by evaluating current priorities and ensuring alignment with personal values and aspirations.

**Goal Realignment Index:**

$$\text{Goal Realignment} = \text{Reflect on Changing Circumstances} + \text{Revised Prioritization}$$

Realign goals by reflecting on changing circumstances and revising prioritization based on evolving needs.

**Resource Optimization Equation:**

$$\text{Resource Optimization} = \text{Resource Redistribution} + \text{Efficient Resource Use}$$

Optimize resources by redistributing them according to changing goals and ensuring efficient utilization.

**Chemical Formula for a Common Learning Neurotransmitter (e.g., Acetylcholine):**

$$C_7H_{16}NO_2$$

Presenting the chemical formula of a common neurotransmitter associated with learning for reference.

**Time Management Adjustments:**

$$\text{Time Management} = \text{Prioritization} + \text{Effective Scheduling}$$

Adjust time management by prioritizing tasks and implementing effective scheduling for goal-oriented activities.

**Continuous Improvement Loop:**

$$\text{Continuous Improvement} = \text{Regular Goal Review} + \text{Strategic Adjustments}$$

Establish a continuous improvement loop by regularly reviewing goals and making strategic adjustments for optimal outcomes.

Incorporating these practical aspects into adjusting goals as needed ensures adaptability and resilience in the pursuit of personal and professional aspirations.

## 8.5 Goal-Setting for Mental Health

Explore practical aspects of goal-setting for mental health:

**Emotional Well-being Equation:**

$$\text{Emotional Well-being} = \text{Positive Affirmations} + \text{Mindful Practices}$$

Enhance emotional well-being by incorporating positive affirmations and engaging in mindful practices regularly.

**Stress Reduction Formula:**

$$\text{Stress Reduction} = \text{Identify Stressors} + \text{Implement Coping Strategies}$$

Reduce stress by identifying stressors and implementing effective coping strategies tailored to individual needs.

**Chemical Formula for a Common Stress Hormone (e.g., Cortisol):**

$$C_{21}H_{30}O_{5}$$

Presenting the chemical formula of a common stress hormone for reference.

**Sleep Quality Optimization System:**

$$\text{Sleep Quality} = \text{Establish Bedtime Routine} + \text{Create Comfortable Sleep Environment}$$

Optimize sleep quality by establishing a bedtime routine and creating a comfortable sleep environment.

**Social Connection Index:**

$$\text{Social Connection} = \text{Meaningful Social Interactions} + \text{Supportive Relationships}$$

Foster mental health through meaningful social interactions and building supportive relationships.

**Chemical Formula for a Common Happiness Neurotransmitter (e.g., Dopamine):**

$$C_{8}H_{11}NO_{2}$$

Presenting the chemical formula of a common neurotransmitter associated with happiness for reference.

**Physical Activity Prescription:**

$$\text{Physical Activity} = \text{Regular Exercise Routine} + \text{Adaptive Movement Practices}$$

Prescribe physical activity for mental health, including a regular exercise routine and adaptive movement practices.

**Mindfulness Integration Equation:**

$$\text{Mindfulness Integration} = \text{Daily Meditation} + \text{Focused Breathing Exercises}$$

Integrate mindfulness into daily life through practices such as daily meditation and focused breathing exercises.

Incorporating these practical aspects into goal-setting for mental health ensures a holistic approach to well-being, promoting a positive and resilient mindset.

## 8.6   Long-Term Vision

Explore practical aspects of cultivating a long-term vision:

**Goal Clarity Formula:**

$$\text{Goal Clarity} = \text{Vision Definition} + \text{SMART Criteria Application}$$

Enhance goal clarity by clearly defining the vision and applying SMART criteria (Specific, Measurable, Achievable, Relevant, Time-Bound).

**Chemical Formula for a Common Motivation Neurotransmitter (e.g., Norepinephrine):**

$$C_8H_{11}NO_3$$

Presenting the chemical formula of a common neurotransmitter associated with motivation for reference.

**Strategic Planning Equation:**

$$\text{Strategic Planning} = \text{Breakdown of Long-Term Goals} + \text{Step-by-Step Action Plan}$$

Create a strategic plan by breaking down long-term goals and developing a step-by-step action plan for execution.

**Adaptability Index:**

$$\text{Adaptability} = \text{Openness to Change} + \text{Feedback Incorporation}$$

Foster adaptability by maintaining openness to change and incorporating feedback into the long-term vision.

**Chemical Formula for a Common Focus Neurotransmitter (e.g., Acetylcholine):**

$$C_7H_{16}NO_2$$

Presenting the chemical formula of a common neurotransmitter associated with focus for reference.

**Visualization Technique:**

$$\text{Visualization} = \text{Imagining Future Success Scenes} + \text{Emotional Connection}$$

Improve goal visualization by imagining scenes of future success and establishing an emotional connection to the long-term vision.

**Resource Allocation System:**

$$\text{Resource Allocation} = \text{Prioritization} + \text{Efficient Resource Utilization}$$

Optimize resource allocation by prioritizing components of the long-term vision and efficiently utilizing available resources.

**Continuous Reflection Loop:**

$$\text{Continuous Reflection} = \text{Regular Progress Evaluation} + \text{Strategic Adjustments}$$

Establish a continuous reflection loop by regularly evaluating progress and making strategic adjustments to align with the long-term vision.

Incorporating these practical aspects into cultivating a long-term vision ensures resilience and focus in the pursuit of meaningful and lasting goals.

## 8.7 Self-Compassion in Goal Pursuit

Explore practical aspects of integrating self-compassion into goal pursuit:

**Compassion Equation:**

$$\text{Compassion} = \text{Self-Love} + \text{Understanding of Imperfection}$$

Cultivate compassion by fostering self-love and embracing an understanding of imperfection in the journey of goal pursuit.

**Chemical Formula for a Common Self-Love Neurotransmitter (e.g., Oxytocin):**

$$C{\cdot}43H{\cdot}66N{\cdot}12O{\cdot}12S{\cdot}2$$

Presenting the chemical formula of a common neurotransmitter associated with feelings of love and compassion for reference.

**Self-Reflection Integration System:**

$$\text{Self-Reflection} = \text{Acknowledge Setbacks} + \text{Learn and Adjust}$$

Integrate self-reflection into goal pursuit by acknowledging setbacks and using them as opportunities to learn and adjust.

**Positive Affirmation Technique:**

$$\text{Positive Affirmation} = \text{Encouraging Self-Talk} + \text{Reframing Negative Thoughts}$$

Incorporate positive affirmations by engaging in encouraging self-talk and reframing negative thoughts with compassion.

**Chemical Formula for a Common Stress-Reducing Neurotransmitter (e.g., Serotonin):**

$$C_{10}H_{12}N_{2}O$$

Presenting the chemical formula of a common neurotransmitter associated with mood regulation and stress reduction for reference.

**Self-Care Equation:**

$$\text{Self-Care} = \text{Prioritize Personal Well-being} + \text{Set Boundaries}$$

Prioritize self-care by emphasizing personal well-being and setting boundaries to maintain balance in goal pursuit.

**Mindfulness in Action System:**

$$\text{Mindfulness} = \text{Present-Moment Awareness} + \text{Non-Judgmental Observation}$$

Practice mindfulness in action by cultivating present-moment awareness and non-judgmental observation in goal-related activities.

**Chemical Formula for a Common Well-being Neurotransmitter (e.g., Endorphins):**

$$C_{30}H_{40}N_{8}O_{8}$$

Presenting the chemical formula of a common neurotransmitter associated with well-being and happiness for reference.

**Continuous Self-Encouragement Loop:**

$$\text{Continuous Self-Encouragement} = \text{Celebrate Small Wins} + \text{Encourage Progress}$$

Establish a continuous self-encouragement loop by celebrating small wins and consistently encouraging progress in goal pursuit.

Incorporating these practical aspects into goal pursuit with self-compassion ensures a supportive and resilient approach to achieving personal and professional aspirations.

# Chapter 9

# Maintaining Mental Health

## 9.1 Preventing Relapse

Explore practical aspects of preventing relapse in maintaining mental health:

**Relapse Prevention Equation:**

$$\text{Relapse Prevention} = \text{Identifying Triggers} + \text{Developing Coping Strategies}$$

Mitigate relapse risks by proactively identifying triggers and developing effective coping strategies.

**Chemical Formula for a Common Stress-Reducing Neurotransmitter (e.g., GABA):**

$$C_4H_9NO_2$$

Presenting the chemical formula of a common neurotransmitter associated with stress reduction for reference.

**Daily Routine Optimization System:**

$$\text{Daily Routine Optimization} = \text{Healthy Habits} + \text{Structured Activities}$$

Optimize daily routines by incorporating healthy habits and structured activities to maintain mental well-being.

**Chemical Formula for a Common Happiness-Inducing Neurotransmitter (e.g., Dopamine):**

$$C_8H_{11}NO_2$$

Presenting the chemical formula of a common neurotransmitter associated with pleasure and happiness for reference.

**Emotional Regulation Formula:**

$$\text{Emotional Regulation} = \text{Mindfulness Practices} + \text{Expressing Emotions}$$

Regulate emotions by engaging in mindfulness practices and expressing emotions in a healthy manner.

**Chemical Formula for a Common Relaxation Neurotransmitter (e.g., Melatonin):**

$$C_{13}H_{16}N_2O_2$$

Presenting the chemical formula of a common neurotransmitter associated with relaxation and sleep for reference.

**Support Network Strengthening Equation:**

$$\text{Support Network Strengthening} = \text{Communicate Openly} + \text{Share Concerns}$$

Strengthen your support network by communicating openly and sharing concerns with trusted individuals.

**Chemical Formula for a Common Bonding Neurotransmitter (e.g., Oxytocin):**

$$C_{43}H_{66}N_{12}O_{12}S_2$$

Presenting the chemical formula of a common neurotransmitter associated with bonding and trust for reference.

**Goal Reinforcement System:**

$$\text{Goal Reinforcement} = \text{Setting Achievable Targets} + \text{Regular Progress Assessment}$$

Reinforce mental health goals by setting achievable targets and regularly assessing progress.

**Chemical Formula for a Common Mood-Stabilizing Neurotransmitter (e.g., Serotonin):**

$$C_{10}H_{12}N_2O$$

Presenting the chemical formula of a common neurotransmitter associated with mood stabilization for reference.

Incorporating these practical aspects into relapse prevention strategies ensures a proactive and resilient approach to maintaining mental health.

## 9.2  Lifestyle Adjustments

Explore practical lifestyle adjustments for maintaining mental health:

**Balanced Lifestyle Equation:**

$$\text{Balanced Lifestyle} = \text{Healthy Diet} + \text{Regular Exercise}$$

Achieve a balanced lifestyle by incorporating a healthy diet and engaging in regular exercise.

**Chemical Formula for a Common Energy-Boosting Neurotransmitter (e.g., Norepinephrine):**

$$C_8H_{11}NO_3$$

Presenting the chemical formula of a common neurotransmitter associated with energy and alertness for reference.

**Quality Sleep Optimization System:**

$$\text{Quality Sleep Optimization} = \text{Establishing a Sleep Routine} + \text{Creating a Comfortable Sleep Environment}$$

Optimize the quality of sleep by establishing a sleep routine and creating a comfortable sleep environment.

**Chemical Formula for a Common Sleep-Inducing Neurotransmitter (e.g., Melatonin):**

$$C_{13}H_{16}N_2O_2$$

Presenting the chemical formula of a common neurotransmitter associated with sleep induction for reference.

**Stress Reduction Technique Integration:**

$$\text{Stress Reduction} = \text{Mindfulness Practices} + \text{Deep Breathing Exercises}$$

Integrate stress reduction techniques by engaging in mindfulness practices and incorporating deep breathing exercises.

**Chemical Formula for a Common Stress-Reducing Neurotransmitter (e.g., GABA):**

$$C_4H_9NO_2$$

Presenting the chemical formula of a common neurotransmitter associated with stress reduction for reference.

**Mindful Technology Use Formula:**

$$\text{Mindful Technology Use} = \text{Digital Detox} + \text{Setting Boundaries}$$

Promote mindful technology use by incorporating digital detox periods and setting boundaries for screen time.

**Chemical Formula for a Common Focus and Attention Neurotransmitter (e.g., Acetylcholine):**

$$C_7H_{16}NO_2$$

Presenting the chemical formula of a common neurotransmitter associated with focus and attention for reference.

**Social Connection Enhancement Equation:**

$$\text{Social Connection Enhancement} = \text{Building Meaningful Relationships} + \text{Joining Social Activities}$$

Enhance social connections by actively building meaningful relationships and participating in social activities.

**Chemical Formula for a Common Bonding Neurotransmitter (e.g., Oxytocin):**

$$C_{43}H_{66}N_{12}O_{12}S_2$$

Presenting the chemical formula of a common neurotransmitter associated with bonding and trust for reference.

Incorporating these practical lifestyle adjustments supports mental health maintenance with an accessible and effective approach.

## 9.3   Regular Check-Ins and Assessments

Explore practical strategies for maintaining mental health through regular check-ins and assessments:

**Personal Wellness Evaluation System:**

$$\text{Personal Wellness} = \text{Emotional Well-being} + \text{Physical Health}$$

Conduct a personal wellness evaluation by considering both emotional well-being and physical health.

**Chemical Formula for a Common Mood-Stabilizing Neurotransmitter (e.g., Serotonin):**

$$C_{10}H_{12}N_2O$$

Presenting the chemical formula of a common neurotransmitter associated with mood stabilization for reference.

**Mood Tracker Equation:**

$$\text{Mood Tracker} = \text{Daily Emotion Reflection} + \text{Identifying Patterns}$$

Utilize a mood tracker by reflecting on daily emotions and identifying patterns for better emotional awareness.

**Chemical Formula for a Common Stress-Reducing Neurotransmitter (e.g., GABA):**

$$C_4H_9NO_2$$

Presenting the chemical formula of a common neurotransmitter associated with stress reduction for reference.

**Activity Log System:**

$$\text{Activity Log} = \text{Daily Tasks} + \text{Leisure Activities}$$

Maintain a balanced activity log by incorporating daily tasks and leisure activities for a sense of accomplishment and enjoyment.

**Chemical Formula for a Common Pleasure-Inducing Neurotransmitter (e.g., Dopamine):**

$$C_8H_{11}NO_2$$

Presenting the chemical formula of a common neurotransmitter associated with pleasure and reward for reference.

**Sleep Quality Assessment Equation:**

$$\text{Sleep Quality Assessment} = \text{Duration} + \text{Restfulness}$$

Assess sleep quality based on both the duration and restfulness of sleep for overall well-being.

**Chemical Formula for a Common Sleep-Inducing Neurotransmitter (e.g., Melatonin):**

$$C_{13}H_{16}N_2O_2$$

Presenting the chemical formula of a common neurotransmitter associated with sleep induction for reference.

**Stress Resilience Scale:**

$$\text{Stress Resilience} = \text{Coping Strategies} + \text{Social Support}$$

Evaluate stress resilience by considering effective coping strategies and the availability of social support.

**Chemical Formula for a Common Bonding Neurotransmitter (e.g., Oxytocin):**

$$C_{43}H_{66}N_{12}O_{12}S_2$$

Presenting the chemical formula of a common neurotransmitter associated with bonding and trust for reference.

Regular check-ins and assessments using these practical strategies contribute to a proactive approach to maintaining mental health.

## 9.4 Long-Term Strategies for Well-being

Explore practical and sustainable strategies for long-term well-being:

**Lifestyle Equation for Resilience:**

$$\text{Resilience} = \text{Healthy Habits} + \text{Adaptability}$$

Build resilience by adopting healthy habits and fostering adaptability to navigate life's challenges.

**Chemical Formula for a Common Stress-Reducing Neurotransmitter (e.g., GABA):**

$$C_4H_9NO_2$$

Presenting the chemical formula of a common neurotransmitter associated with stress reduction for reference.

**Emotional Intelligence Framework:**

$$\text{Emotional Intelligence} = \text{Self-Awareness} + \text{Empathy}$$

Develop emotional intelligence by enhancing self-awareness and fostering empathy for better interpersonal relationships.

**Chemical Formula for a Common Empathy-Inducing Neurotransmitter (e.g., Endorphins):**

$$C_{30}H_{31}N_3O_7$$

Presenting the chemical formula of a common neurotransmitter associated with empathy and pleasure for reference.

**Holistic Self-Care Equation:**

$$\text{Holistic Self-Care} = \text{Physical Health} + \text{Mental Wellness}$$

Prioritize holistic self-care by addressing both physical health and mental wellness for comprehensive well-being.

**Chemical Formula for a Common Well-being Neurotransmitter (e.g., Serotonin):**

$$C_{10}H_{12}N_2O$$

Presenting the chemical formula of a common neurotransmitter associated with mood stabilization and well-being for reference.

**Personal Growth Model:**

$$\text{Personal Growth} = \text{Continuous Learning} + \text{Reflection}$$

Foster personal growth through continuous learning and reflective practices for ongoing development.

**Chemical Formula for a Common Learning-Inducing Neurotransmitter (e.g., Glutamate):**

$$C_5H_9NO_4$$

Presenting the chemical formula of a common neurotransmitter associated with learning and memory for reference.

**Social Connection Framework:**

$$\text{Social Connection} = \text{Quality Relationships} + \text{Community Engagement}$$

Cultivate social connection by nurturing quality relationships and actively engaging with the community.

**Chemical Formula for a Common Bonding Neurotransmitter (e.g., Oxytocin):**

$$C_{43}H_{66}N_{12}O_{12}S_2$$

Presenting the chemical formula of a common neurotransmitter associated with bonding and trust for reference.

Adopting these long-term strategies promotes sustained well-being and contributes to a fulfilling and meaningful life.

## 9.5    Creating a Wellness Plan

Crafting a wellness plan involves practical and effective strategies:

**Wellness Equation:**

$$Wellness = Balanced\ Lifestyle + Self\text{-}Care$$

Achieve overall wellness by maintaining a balanced lifestyle and prioritizing self-care.

**Chemical Formula for a Common Well-being Neurotransmitter (e.g., Dopamine):**

$$C_8H_{11}NO_2$$

Presenting the chemical formula of a common neurotransmitter associated with pleasure and reward for reference.

**Daily Routine Optimization:**

$$Optimized\ Routine = Quality\ Sleep + Nutrient\text{-}Rich\ Diet + Physical\ Activity$$

Optimize your daily routine by ensuring quality sleep, maintaining a nutrient-rich diet, and incorporating regular physical activity.

**Chemical Formula for a Common Sleep-Inducing Neurotransmitter (e.g., Melatonin):**

$$C_{13}H_{16}N_2O_2$$

Presenting the chemical formula of a common neurotransmitter associated with sleep regulation for reference.

**Mindful Stress Management:**

$$Stress\ Management = Mindfulness + Breathing\ Techniques$$

Manage stress mindfully by incorporating mindfulness practices and effective breathing techniques.

**Chemical Formula for a Common Relaxation Neurotransmitter (e.g., GABA):**

$$C_4H_9NO_2$$

Presenting the chemical formula of a common neurotransmitter associated with relaxation and calmness for reference.

**Emotional Resilience Blueprint:**

$$\text{Emotional Resilience} = \text{Emotional Awareness} + \text{Coping Strategies}$$

Build emotional resilience through heightened emotional awareness and adaptive coping strategies.

**Chemical Formula for a Common Stress-Reducing Neurotransmitter (e.g., Serotonin):**

$$C_{10}H_{12}N_2O$$

Presenting the chemical formula of a common neurotransmitter associated with mood stabilization for reference.

**Social Connection Matrix:**

$$\text{Social Connection} = \text{Quality Relationships} + \text{Active Social Engagement}$$

Enhance social connection by nurturing quality relationships and actively engaging in social activities.

**Chemical Formula for a Common Social-Bonding Neurotransmitter (e.g., Oxytocin):**

$$C_{43}H_{66}N_{12}O_{12}S_2$$

Presenting the chemical formula of a common neurotransmitter associated with social bonding for reference.

Crafting and adhering to a wellness plan incorporating these elements contributes to lasting mental health.

## 9.6 Tracking Progress

Efficiently track your mental health progress with practical strategies:

**Goal Achievement Formula:**

$$\text{Goal Achievement} = \text{Actionable Steps} + \text{Consistent Effort}$$

Successfully achieve your goals by breaking them into actionable steps and maintaining consistent effort.

**Chemical Formula for a Common Motivation Neurotransmitter (e.g., Norepinephrine):**

$$C_8H_{11}NO_3$$

Presenting the chemical formula of a common neurotransmitter associated with motivation for reference.

**Quantifiable Metrics for Well-being:**

$$\text{Well-being Metrics} = \text{Mood Ratings} + \text{Energy Levels} + \text{Sleep Quality}$$

Quantify your well-being by assessing mood ratings, energy levels, and sleep quality regularly.

**Chemical Formula for a Common Energy-Boosting Neurotransmitter (e.g., Adenosine Triphosphate):**

$$C_{10}H_{16}N_5O_{13}P_3$$

Presenting the chemical formula of a common molecule associated with cellular energy transfer for reference.

**Habit Formation Equation:**

$$\text{Habit Formation} = \text{Cue Recognition} + \text{Routine Consistency} + \text{Reward Satisfaction}$$

Form lasting habits by recognizing cues, maintaining routine consistency, and finding satisfaction in the rewards.

**Chemical Formula for a Common Learning-Associated Neurotransmitter (e.g., Glutamate):**

$$C_5H_9NO_4$$

Presenting the chemical formula of a common neurotransmitter associated with learning and memory for reference.

**Mindfulness Checkpoints:**

$$\text{Mindfulness Checkpoints} = \text{Daily Reflection} + \text{Gratitude Practice}$$

Stay mindful with daily reflection and incorporating gratitude practices into your routine.

**Chemical Formula for a Common Calming Neurotransmitter (e.g., Gamma-Aminobutyric Acid):**

$$C_4H_9NO_2$$

Presenting the chemical formula of a common neurotransmitter associated with calming effects for reference.

**Personal Growth Assessment:**

$$\text{Personal Growth} = \text{Challenges Overcome} + \text{New Skills Acquired}$$

Assess personal growth by reflecting on challenges overcome and new skills acquired.

**Chemical Formula for a Common Pleasure-Inducing Neurotransmitter (e.g., Endorphins):**

$$C_{29}H_{38}N_2O_9$$

Presenting the chemical formula of a common neurotransmitter associated with pleasure and pain relief for reference.

Implement these tracking strategies to witness and celebrate your mental health progress effectively.

## 9.7  Adapting to Life Changes

Efficiently adapt to life changes with practical strategies:

**Resilience Formula:**

$$\text{Resilience} = \text{Adaptability} + \text{Mindset}$$

Build resilience by enhancing adaptability and cultivating a positive mindset.

**Chemical Formula for a Common Stress-Reducing Neurotransmitter (e.g., Serotonin):**

$$C_{10}H_{12}N_2O$$

Presenting the chemical formula of a common neurotransmitter associated with mood regulation and stress reduction for reference.

**Flow State Equation:**

$$\text{Flow State} = \text{Challenge Level} - \text{Skill Level}$$

Achieve a flow state by balancing the challenge level with your skill level.

**Chemical Formula for a Common Relaxation-Inducing Neurotransmitter (e.g., Dopamine):**

$$C_8H_{11}NO_2$$

Presenting the chemical formula of a common neurotransmitter associated with relaxation and reward for reference.

**Adaptation Strategies:**

$$\text{Adaptation Strategies} = \text{Problem-Solving} + \text{Flexible Thinking}$$

Effectively adapt by employing problem-solving skills and maintaining flexible thinking.

**Chemical Formula for a Common Memory-Enhancing Neurotransmitter (e.g., Acetylcholine):**

$$C_7H_{16}NO_2$$

Presenting the chemical formula of a common neurotransmitter associated with memory and learning for reference.

**Emotional Intelligence Formula:**

$$\text{Emotional Intelligence} = \text{Self-Awareness} + \text{Social Awareness} + \text{Emotional Regulation}$$

Boost emotional intelligence by cultivating self-awareness, social awareness, and emotional regulation.

**Chemical Formula for a Common Motivation Neurotransmitter (e.g., Norepinephrine):**

$$C_8H_{11}NO_3$$

Presenting the chemical formula of a common neurotransmitter associated with motivation for reference.

**Mindfulness in Change:**

$$\text{Mindfulness in Change} = \text{Present Moment Awareness} + \text{Acceptance}$$

Practice mindfulness in change by embracing present moment awareness and fostering acceptance.

**Chemical Formula for a Common Focus-Inducing Neurotransmitter (e.g., Noradrenaline):**

$$C_8H_{11}NO_3$$

Presenting the chemical formula of a common neurotransmitter associated with focus and attention for reference.

Implement these strategies to smoothly adapt to life changes and maintain your mental well-being effectively.

# Chapter 10

# Fostering Resilience

## 10.1  Resilience in the Face of Challenges

Navigate challenges with resilience through practical strategies:

**Resilience Equation:**

$$Resilience = Adaptability + Positive\ Mindset$$

Cultivate resilience by enhancing adaptability and fostering a positive mindset.

**Chemical Formula for a Common Stress-Reducing Neurotransmitter (e.g., Serotonin):**

$$C_{10}H_{12}N_2O$$

Presenting the chemical formula of a common neurotransmitter associated with mood regulation and stress reduction for reference.

**Growth Mindset Formula:**

$$Growth\ Mindset = Learning + Persistence$$

Develop a growth mindset by prioritizing continuous learning and persistent effort.

**Chemical Formula for a Common Relaxation-Inducing Neurotransmitter (e.g., Dopamine):**

$$C_8H_{11}NO_2$$

Presenting the chemical formula of a common neurotransmitter associated with relaxation and reward for reference.

**Coping Mechanism Equation:**

$$\text{Coping Mechanism} = \text{Awareness} + \text{Healthy Outlets}$$

Enhance coping mechanisms by cultivating self-awareness and engaging in healthy outlets.

**Chemical Formula for a Common Memory-Enhancing Neurotransmitter (e.g., Acetylcholine):**

$$C_7H_{16}NO_2$$

Presenting the chemical formula of a common neurotransmitter associated with memory and learning for reference.

**Resilience-Building Strategies:**

$$\text{Resilience-Building Strategies} = \text{Problem-Solving} + \text{Support Systems}$$

Strengthen resilience with effective problem-solving skills and robust support systems.

**Chemical Formula for a Common Motivation Neurotransmitter (e.g., Norepinephrine):**

$$C_8H_{11}NO_3$$

Presenting the chemical formula of a common neurotransmitter associated with motivation for reference.

**Mindfulness in Challenges:**

$$\text{Mindfulness in Challenges} = \text{Present Moment Awareness} + \text{Acceptance}$$

Practice mindfulness in the face of challenges by embracing present moment awareness and fostering acceptance.

**Chemical Formula for a Common Focus-Inducing Neurotransmitter (e.g., Noradrenaline):**

$$C_8H_{11}NO_3$$

Presenting the chemical formula of a common neurotransmitter associated with focus and attention for reference.

Implement these strategies to foster resilience and navigate challenges with strength and adaptability.

## 10.2  Learning from Setbacks

Embrace setbacks as opportunities for growth with practical strategies:

**Resilience Formula:**

$$\text{Resilience} = \text{Learning from Setbacks} + \text{Adaptability}$$

Boost resilience by actively learning from setbacks and cultivating adaptability.

**Chemical Equation for Resilience (Symbolic Representation):**

$$\text{Res} \xrightarrow{\text{Setbacks}} \text{Growth}$$

Symbolically represent the transformative process of setbacks leading to personal growth.

**Mindset Shift Formula:**

$$\text{Mindset Shift} = \text{Reflection} + \text{Positive Reframing}$$

Initiate a mindset shift by reflecting on setbacks and reframing them positively.

**Chemical Reaction for Positive Reframing:**

$$\text{Negativity} + \text{Reflection} \xrightarrow{\text{Positive Reframing}} \text{Optimism}$$

Conceptually illustrate the chemical reaction where negativity, through reflection, transforms into optimism.

**Adaptability Enhancement Equation:**

$$\text{Adaptability Enhancement} = \text{Flexible Thinking} + \text{Resourcefulness}$$

Enhance adaptability by fostering flexible thinking and resourcefulness.

**Chemical Formula for Flexible Thinking (Symbolic Representation):**

$$C_6H_{12}O_6$$

Symbolically represent the chemical formula for a compound associated with cognitive flexibility.

**Turning Setbacks into Opportunities Strategy:**

$$\text{Turning Setbacks into Opportunities} = \text{Creativity} + \text{Solution-Focused Thinking}$$

Transform setbacks into opportunities by channeling creativity and adopting a solution-focused mindset.

**Chemical Formula for Solution-Focused Thinking (Symbolic Representation):**

$$\text{Solu} \xrightarrow{\text{Setbacks}} \text{Opportunity}$$

Symbolically represent the process where setbacks lead to opportunities through solution-focused thinking.

**Learning Resilience from Nature Principle:**

$$\text{Nature Resilience} = \text{Adaptation} + \text{Regeneration}$$

Draw inspiration from nature's resilience by observing its principles of adaptation and regeneration.

**Chemical Equation for Regeneration:**

$$\text{Stagnation} \xrightarrow{\text{Adaptation}} \text{Renewal}$$

Conceptually illustrate the chemical reaction where stagnation, through adaptation, leads to renewal.

Incorporate these practical strategies to learn from setbacks, fostering resilience and personal growth.

## 10.3  Cultivating a Positive Mindset

Nurture a positive mindset with actionable strategies:

**Mindset Cultivation Formula:**

$$\text{Positive Mindset} = \text{Gratitude} + \text{Affirmations} + \text{Mindfulness}$$

Cultivate a positive mindset by embracing gratitude, affirmations, and mindfulness.

**Chemical Equation for Gratitude Expression:**

$$\text{Negativity} + \text{Gratitude} \xrightarrow{\text{Expression}} \text{Positivity}$$

Express gratitude to transform negativity into positivity, creating a chemical reaction.

**Affirmation Empowerment Formula:**

$$\text{Empowerment} = \text{Self-Affirmation} + \text{Positive Self-Talk}$$

Empower yourself through self-affirmation and positive self-talk.

**Chemical Formula for Positive Self-Talk (Symbolic Representation):**

$$\text{Self} \xrightarrow{\text{Positive Self-Talk}} \text{Confidence}$$

Symbolically represent the process where positive self-talk enhances self-confidence.

**Mindfulness Integration Equation:**

$$\text{Mindfulness Integration} = \text{Present-Moment Awareness} + \text{Non-Judgmental Observation}$$

Integrate mindfulness by fostering present-moment awareness and non-judgmental observation.

**Chemical Reaction for Present-Moment Awareness:**

$$\text{Past} + \text{Present} \xrightarrow{\text{Awareness}} \text{Mindful Presence}$$

Conceptually illustrate the chemical reaction where awareness of past and present leads to mindful presence.

**Positivity Amplification Strategy:**

$$\text{Positivity Amplification} = \text{Kindness} + \text{Joy Sharing}$$

Amplify positivity by practicing kindness and sharing moments of joy.

**Chemical Equation for Joy Sharing:**

$$\text{Joy} \xrightarrow{\text{Sharing}} \text{Multiply}$$

Illustrate the process where sharing joy multiplies the positive impact, akin to a chemical reaction.

**Neuroscience of Positivity Principle:**

$$\text{Neuroplasticity} = \text{Positive Thoughts} + \text{Repetition}$$

Harness neuroplasticity by cultivating positive thoughts through repetition.

**Chemical Formula for Repetition (Symbolic Representation):**

$$\text{Neuro} \xrightarrow{\text{Repetition}} \text{Growth}$$

Symbolically represent the process where neuroplasticity, through repetition, leads to personal growth.

Incorporate these practical strategies to cultivate a positive mindset, fostering resilience and well-being.

## 10.4 Adversity as a Catalyst for Growth

Discover the transformative power of adversity with actionable insights:

**Resilience Growth Formula:**

$$\text{Resilience} = \text{Adversity} + \text{Learning} + \text{Adaptation}$$

Harness adversity as a catalyst for resilience by embracing a continual cycle of learning and adaptation.

**Chemical Equation for Learning from Adversity:**

$$\text{Challenge} \xrightarrow{\text{Reflection}} \text{Wisdom}$$

Reflect on challenges to extract wisdom, initiating a chemical-like transformation.

**Adaptation Mechanism:**

$$\text{Adaptation} = \text{Flexibility} + \text{Positive Reframing}$$

Develop resilience through adaptation, blending flexibility and positive reframing.

**Chemical Reaction for Positive Reframing:**

$$\text{Negative} \xrightarrow{\text{Reframe}} \text{Positive Outlook}$$

Reframe negative experiences, triggering a chemical reaction that fosters a positive outlook.

**Growth Mindset Principle:**

$$\text{Growth Mindset} = \text{Challenge Acceptance} + \text{Effort}$$

Cultivate a growth mindset by accepting challenges and putting in effort.

**Chemical Formula for Effort (Symbolic Representation):**

$$\text{Mindset} \xrightarrow{\text{Effort}} \text{Growth}$$

Symbolically represent the process where effort, within a growth mindset, leads to personal growth.

**Resilience Catalyst Strategy:**

$$\text{Catalyst} = \text{Optimism} + \text{Social Support}$$

Optimism and social support act as catalysts, accelerating the resilience-building process.

**Chemical Equation for Social Support:**

$$\text{Isolation} \xrightarrow{\text{Support}} \text{Strength}$$

Highlight the transformative effect where social support converts isolation into strength.

**Neuroscience of Resilience Activation:**

$$\text{Neural Rewiring} = \text{Challenge Response} + \text{Positive Affirmation}$$

Activate neural rewiring through a positive response to challenges and affirmations.

**Chemical Formula for Affirmation (Symbolic Representation):**

$$\text{Neural} \xrightarrow{\text{Affirmation}} \text{Strength}$$

Symbolically represent the process where neural rewiring, via affirmation, leads to inner strength.

Embrace adversity as a catalyst, unlocking the potential for profound personal growth and resilience.

## 10.5  Building Emotional Resilience

Unlock the power of emotional resilience with practical strategies:

**Emotional Resilience Framework:**

$$\text{Emotional Resilience} = \text{Self-awareness} + \text{Emotional Regulation} + \text{Positive Coping}$$

Enhance emotional resilience by integrating self-awareness, emotional regulation, and positive coping mechanisms.

**Chemical Equation for Self-awareness:**

$$\text{Reflection} \xrightarrow{\text{Awareness}} \text{Emotional Intelligence}$$

Initiate a chemical-like reaction where reflective practices lead to heightened emotional intelligence.

**Emotional Regulation Formula:**

$$\text{Emotion Regulation} = \text{Mindfulness} + \text{Expressive Outlet}$$

Regulate emotions by combining mindfulness practices with expressive outlets.

**Chemical Reaction for Expressive Outlet:**

$$\text{Emotion} \xrightarrow{\text{Expression}} \text{Catharsis}$$

Express emotions to catalyze a cathartic release, fostering emotional well-being.

**Positive Coping Strategy:**

$$\text{Positive Coping} = \text{Adaptability} + \text{Social Connection}$$

Cultivate positive coping mechanisms through adaptability and fostering social connections.

**Chemical Formula for Social Connection:**

$$\text{Isolation} \xrightarrow{\text{Connection}} \text{Strength}$$

Transform isolation into strength through the alchemy of social connections.

**Neurochemistry of Emotional Resilience:**

$$\text{Neurotransmitter Balance} = \text{Positive Thinking} + \text{Mindful Breathing}$$

Balance neurotransmitters by incorporating positive thinking and mindful breathing practices.

**Chemical Equation for Positive Thinking:**

$$\text{Negative Thoughts} \xrightarrow{\text{Positivity}} \text{Neurotransmitter Balance}$$

Alchemize negative thoughts into a balanced neurochemistry through the power of positivity.

**Mindfulness Integration:**

$$\text{Mindfulness} = \text{Present-moment Awareness} + \text{Non-judgmental Observation}$$

Immerse in mindfulness through present-moment awareness and non-judgmental observation.

**Chemical Reaction for Mindfulness:**

$$\text{Stress} \xrightarrow{\text{Mindfulness}} \text{Calmness}$$

Experience a chemical transformation where mindfulness dismantles stress, fostering a sense of calmness.

Empower yourself with the tools to build emotional resilience, incorporating self-awareness, regulation, and positive coping strategies.

# 10.6  Resilience in Daily Life

Discover the essence of resilience in your daily life with practical equations:

**Daily Resilience Formula:**

$$\text{Resilience} = \text{Adaptability} + \text{Mindful Response}$$

Cultivate resilience by blending adaptability with a mindful response to life's challenges.

**Adaptability Equation:**

$$\text{Adaptability} = \text{Open-mindedness} + \text{Flexibility}$$

Enhance adaptability through the combination of open-mindedness and flexibility.

**Chemical Reaction for Open-mindedness:**

$$\text{Preconceptions} \xrightarrow{\text{Open-mindedness}} \text{Possibilities}$$

Transform preconceptions into a world of possibilities through the alchemy of open-mindedness.

**Flexibility Formula:**

$$\text{Flexibility} = \text{Acceptance} + \text{Creative Problem-solving}$$

Embrace flexibility by integrating acceptance and creative problem-solving into your mindset.

**Chemical Equation for Acceptance:**

$$\text{Resistance} \xrightarrow{\text{Acceptance}} \text{Adaptation}$$

Convert resistance into adaptation through the transformative power of acceptance.

**Mindful Response Strategy:**

$$\text{Mindful Response} = \text{Present Awareness} + \text{Pause and Reflect}$$

Craft a mindful response by combining present awareness with intentional pauses for reflection.

**Chemical Reaction for Present Awareness:**

$$\text{Distraction} \xrightarrow{\text{Awareness}} \text{Clarity}$$

Turn distractions into moments of clarity through the chemical process of heightened awareness.

**Reflection Catalyst:**

$$\text{Pause and Reflect} = \text{Self-discovery} + \text{Continuous Improvement}$$

Initiate a transformative pause for reflection, leading to self-discovery and a commitment to continuous improvement.

**Chemical Equation for Continuous Improvement:**

$$\text{Status Quo} \xrightarrow{\text{Improvement}} \text{Growth}$$

Elevate beyond the status quo by fostering a continuous improvement mindset, sparking personal growth.

Empower your daily life with the resilience formula, integrating adaptability and a mindful response into your routine.

## 10.7   Adapting to Change

Unlock the secrets of adapting to change with practical equations:

**Change Adaptation Formula:**

$$\text{Change Adaptation} = \text{Flexibility} + \text{Positive Outlook}$$

Navigate change by combining flexibility with a positive outlook to foster resilience.

**Flexibility Equation:**

$$\text{Flexibility} = \text{Open-mindedness} + \text{Versatility}$$

Cultivate flexibility by merging open-mindedness with versatile responses to varying situations.

**Chemical Transformation of Open-mindedness:**

$$\text{Preconceptions} \xrightarrow{\text{Open-mindedness}} \text{Possibilities}$$

Transmute preconceptions into a realm of possibilities through the alchemical process of open-mindedness.

**Versatility Equation:**

$$\text{Versatility} = \text{Adaptability} + \text{Skill Diversification}$$

Enhance versatility through the synergy of adaptability and the diversification of skills.

**Chemical Fusion for Skill Diversification:**

$$\text{Specialization} \xrightarrow{\text{Skill Diversification}} \text{Versatility}$$

Blend specialized skills into a versatile toolkit, unlocking a more adaptable approach to change.

**Positive Outlook Strategy:**

$$\text{Positive Outlook} = \text{Gratitude} + \text{Focus on Solutions}$$

Embrace change with a positive outlook by infusing gratitude and a solution-focused mindset.

**Chemical Reaction for Gratitude:**

$$\text{Complaining} \xrightarrow{\text{Gratitude}} \text{Appreciation}$$

Metamorphose complaining into appreciation through the transformative power of gratitude.

**Solution-Focused Mindset Catalyst:**

$$\text{Focus on Solutions} = \text{Problem Analysis} + \text{Action Planning}$$

Tackle change head-on with a solution-focused mindset by analyzing problems and crafting strategic action plans.

**Chemical Synthesis for Action Planning:**

$$\text{Uncertainty} \xrightarrow{\text{Action Planning}} \text{Empowered Response}$$

Convert uncertainty into empowered responses through the chemical synthesis of proactive action planning.

Equip yourself with the adaptation formula, merging flexibility and a positive outlook to thrive amidst change.

# Chapter 11

# Spirituality and Inner Strength

## 11.1 Exploring Personal Beliefs

Embark on a journey of self-discovery and inner strength through the exploration of personal beliefs.

**Belief Exploration Framework:**

$$\text{Personal Beliefs} = \text{Reflection} + \text{Questioning}$$

Uncover the depths of personal beliefs by combining thoughtful reflection with curious questioning.

**Chemical Reaction of Reflection:**

$$\text{Uncertainty} \xrightarrow{\text{Reflection}} \text{Clarity}$$

Transform uncertainty into clarity through the alchemy of introspective reflection.

**Questioning Catalyst:**

$$\text{Questioning} = \text{Curiosity} + \text{Open-minded Inquiry}$$

Ignite the flame of exploration by infusing curiosity and open-minded inquiry into your questioning.

**Chemical Fusion for Open-minded Inquiry:**

$$\text{Dogma} \xrightarrow{\text{Open-minded Inquiry}} \text{Expansive Understanding}$$

Break free from dogma, allowing open-minded inquiry to distill an expansive understanding of personal beliefs.

**Alignment Equation:**

$$\text{Alignment} = \text{Values} + \text{Actions}$$

Forge inner strength by aligning personal beliefs with values and translating them into purposeful actions.

**Chemical Synthesis for Values-Actions Alignment:**

$$\text{Misalignment} \xrightarrow{\text{Values-Actions Alignment}} \text{Empowerment}$$

Harmonize values and actions, transcending misalignment to empower your journey of inner strength.

**Resilience Catalyst:**

$$\text{Resilience} = \text{Acceptance} + \text{Adaptability}$$

Build resilience by combining the power of acceptance with the ability to adapt to evolving beliefs.

**Chemical Reaction for Acceptance:**

$$\text{Resistance} \xrightarrow{\text{Acceptance}} \text{Resilience}$$

Metamorphose resistance into resilience through the chemical reaction of embracing acceptance.

Embark on the path of spirituality and inner strength through the dynamic interplay of reflection, questioning, alignment, and resilience.

## 11.2   Connecting with Inner Strength

Embark on a transformative journey to connect with your inner strength effortlessly.

**Inner Strength Activation:**

$$\text{Inner Strength} = \text{Self-Awareness} \times \text{Self-Compassion}$$

Ignite your inner strength by multiplying self-awareness with the nurturing power of self-compassion.

**Chemical Fusion for Self-Awareness:**

$$\text{Uncertainty} \xrightarrow{\text{Self-Reflection}} \text{Clarity}$$

Transform uncertainty into clarity through the alchemy of self-reflection, unraveling the layers of self-awareness.

**Self-Compassion Equation:**

$$\text{Self-Compassion} = \text{Kindness} + \text{Acceptance}$$

Fuel your inner strength with the potent blend of kindness and acceptance within the realm of self-compassion.

**Chemical Alchemy for Acceptance:**

$$\text{Resistance} \xrightarrow{\text{Acceptance}} \text{Empowerment}$$

Transmute resistance into empowerment by embracing the transformative force of acceptance.

**Mind-Body Synergy:**

$$\text{Mind-Body Synergy} = \text{Mental Resilience} + \text{Physical Vitality}$$

Forge a powerful connection with your inner strength by uniting mental resilience with physical vitality.

**Chemical Fusion for Resilience:**

$$\text{Challenges} \xrightarrow{\text{Resilience}} \text{Growth}$$

Metabolize challenges into personal growth through the chemical fusion of resilience, fostering mind-body synergy.

**Flow State Activation:**

$$\text{Flow State} = \text{Passion} \times \text{Focus}$$

Attain a state of effortless connection with inner strength by multiplying passion with unwavering focus.

**Chemical Reaction for Passion:**

$$\text{Stagnation} \xrightarrow{\text{Passion}} \text{Dynamic Energy}$$

Elevate from stagnation to dynamic energy through the catalytic power of embracing passion.

Connect deeply with your inner strength through the harmonious interplay of self-awareness, self-compassion, mind-body synergy, and the dynamic energy of passion.

# 11.3   Finding Meaning and Purpose

Uncover the essence of your existence effortlessly by delving into the realm of meaning and purpose.

**Equation for Meaning:**

$$\text{Meaning} = \text{Passion} + \text{Contributions}$$

Discover profound meaning by combining the fuel of passion with the impactful energy of making meaningful contributions.

**Chemical Fusion for Passion:**

$$\text{Stagnation} \xrightarrow{\text{Passion}} \text{Dynamic Energy}$$

Elevate from stagnation to dynamic energy through the catalytic power of embracing passion.

**Formula for Contributions:**

$$\text{Contributions} = \text{Skills} \times \text{Service}$$

Unleash the transformative potential of contributions by multiplying your unique skills with a heart dedicated to service.

**Chemical Bonding for Service:**

$$\text{Self-Service} + \text{Community-Service} \xrightarrow{\text{Meaningful Impact}} \text{Purpose}$$

Forge a meaningful impact by bonding self-service and community-service, giving birth to a profound sense of purpose.

**Existential Equation:**

$$\text{Existence} = \text{Being} + \text{Becoming}$$

Navigate the vast landscape of existence by harmonizing the essence of being with the perpetual journey of becoming.

**Chemical Transformation for Becoming:**

$$\text{Potential} \xrightarrow{\text{Continuous Growth}} \text{Unlimited Possibilities}$$

Transmute potential into unlimited possibilities through the chemical transformation of continuous growth.

**Mind-Body Alignment:**

$$\text{Mind-Body Alignment} = \text{Alignment with Values} + \text{Physical Well-being}$$

Attain mind-body alignment by syncing your actions with core values and nurturing physical well-being.

**Chemical Harmony for Values:**

$$\text{Confusion} \xrightarrow{\text{Clarity of Values}} \text{Aligned Choices}$$

Clear the fog of confusion by infusing clarity into your values, paving the way for aligned choices.

Embark on a purposeful journey of self-discovery, where meaning and purpose intertwine seamlessly through passion, contributions, and the alignment of being and becoming.

## 11.4  Spirituality and Mental Health

Unlock the powerful connection between spirituality and mental well-being, paving the way for enduring inner strength.

**Equation for Spiritual Resilience:**

$$\text{Spiritual Resilience} = \text{Belief in Transcendence} + \text{Mindfulness}$$

Enhance your mental fortitude by combining a belief in transcendence with the practice of mindfulness.

**Chemical Fusion for Transcendence:**

$$\text{Materialism} \xrightarrow{\text{Spiritual Beliefs}} \text{Transcendent Outlook}$$

Shift from a materialistic perspective to a transcendent outlook through the alchemical process of embracing spiritual beliefs.

**Formula for Mindfulness:**

$$\text{Mindfulness} = \text{Present Moment Awareness} + \text{Non-judgmental Acceptance}$$

Cultivate mental clarity by merging present moment awareness with non-judgmental acceptance.

**Chemical Balance for Present Moment Awareness:**

$$\text{Distraction} \xrightarrow{\text{Mindful Focus}} \text{Present Mind}$$

Dissolve distractions with mindful focus, bringing your mind into the serene embrace of the present moment.

**Psychological Alchemy:**

$$\text{Negative Thoughts} \xrightarrow{\text{Spiritual Reflection}} \text{Positive Mindset}$$

Transform negative thoughts into positive resilience through the alchemical process of spiritual reflection.

**Inner Harmony Equation:**

$$\text{Inner Harmony} = \text{Connection with Higher Self} + \text{Self-Compassion}$$

Attain inner harmony by nurturing a connection with your higher self and showering yourself with self-compassion.

**Chemical Synthesis for Self-Compassion:**

$$\text{Self-Criticism} \xrightarrow{\text{Self-Compassion Practices}} \text{Inner Nurturing}$$

Break free from self-criticism through the transformative power of self-compassion practices, fostering inner nurturing.

Merge the profound impact of spiritual beliefs and mindfulness to foster spiritual resilience, promoting mental health and fortifying your inner strength.

## 11.5 Practices for Inner Peace

Discover tangible practices that usher in inner peace, seamlessly merging spirituality with your daily life.

**Equation for Tranquility:**

$$\text{Tranquility} = \text{Mindful Breathing} + \text{Gratitude Practices}$$

Achieve a state of calm by blending mindful breathing techniques with the transformative power of gratitude practices.

**Chemical Fusion for Mindful Breathing:**

$$\text{Shallow Breathing} \xrightarrow{\text{Mindful Breath Awareness}} \text{Deep Serenity}$$

Transition from shallow breathing to a deep serenity through the alchemical process of mindful breath awareness.

**Formula for Gratitude Practices:**

$$\text{Gratitude Practices} = \text{Daily Reflections} + \text{Acts of Kindness}$$

Elevate your spirit with gratitude practices, intertwining daily reflections and acts of kindness.

**Chemical Balance for Daily Reflections:**

$$\text{Negative Thoughts} \xrightarrow{\text{Gratitude Reflection}} \text{Positive Mindset}$$

Alchemy of the mind: Convert negative thoughts into a positive mindset through the transformative power of gratitude reflection.

**Psychological Alchemy:**

$$\text{Stressful Thoughts} \xrightarrow{\text{Mindful Release}} \text{Inner Calm}$$

Alleviate stressful thoughts by mindfully releasing them, paving the way for profound inner calm.

**Inner Harmony Equation:**

$$\text{Inner Harmony} = \text{Connection with Nature} + \text{Mindful Presence}$$

Attain inner harmony by fostering a connection with nature and embracing mindful presence.

**Chemical Synthesis for Connection with Nature:**

$$\text{Urban Stress} \xrightarrow{\text{Nature Interaction}} \text{Soulful Serenity}$$

Counter urban stress with the alchemical essence of nature interaction, leading to soulful serenity.

Merge the science of mindful breathing, gratitude practices, and nature connection to cultivate inner peace, making spirituality an integral part of your everyday well-being.

## 11.6 Mind-Body-Spirit Connection

Embark on a transformative journey as we explore the dynamic interplay of the mind, body, and spirit.

**Unified Field Equation:**

$$\text{Mind-Body-Spirit Harmony} = \text{Mental Resilience} + \text{Physical Vitality} + \text{Soulful Alignment}$$

Achieve profound harmony by balancing mental resilience, physical vitality, and soulful alignment in the unified field of your being.

**Biochemical Symphony:**

$$\text{Stress Hormones} \xrightarrow{\text{Mindful Practices}} \text{Calm Neurotransmitters}$$

Conduct a biochemical symphony within, transforming stress hormones into calm neurotransmitters through the practice of mindfulness.

**Energetic Resonance Formula:**

$$\text{Positive Thoughts} \xrightarrow{\text{Body Movement}} \text{Elevated Spiritual Vibration}$$

Elevate your spiritual vibration by translating positive thoughts into kinetic energy through intentional body movement.

**Quantum Entanglement of Emotions:**

$$\text{Joyful Emotions} \xleftrightarrow{\text{Spiritual Practices}} \text{Enhanced Physical Well-being}$$

Experience the quantum entanglement of emotions, where joyful feelings enhance physical well-being through dedicated spiritual practices.

**Molecular Alchemy:**

$$\text{Harmonized Breathing} \xrightarrow{\text{Spiritual Reflection}} \text{Cellular Regeneration}$$

Undergo molecular alchemy by harmonizing your breath and engaging in spiritual reflection, fostering cellular regeneration and renewal.

**Harmony of Chakras:**

$$\text{Balanced Chakras} \xleftrightarrow{\text{Holistic Wellness}} \text{Mind-Body-Spirit Equilibrium}$$

Attain mind-body-spirit equilibrium as you align and balance your chakras through holistic wellness practices.

**Quantum Leap into Wholeness:**

$$\text{Fragmented Existence} \xrightarrow{\text{Mind-Body-Spirit Integration}} \text{Holistic Wholeness}$$

Make a quantum leap into holistic wholeness, transcending fragmented existence through the integration of mind, body, and spirit.

Immerse yourself in the transformative power of the mind-body-spirit connection, embracing a harmonious existence that resonates with the essence of your being.

# 11.7 Transcending Adversity

Embark on a journey of resilience and inner fortitude, transcending adversity with practical wisdom.

**Resilience Formula:**

$$\text{Adversity} \xrightarrow{\text{Spiritual Strength}} \text{Personal Growth}$$

Transform adversity into a catalyst for personal growth, fortified by the strength derived from spiritual practices.

**Quantum Mind-Shift Equation:**

$$\text{Challenges} \xrightarrow{\text{Positive Perspective}} \text{Quantum Mind-Shift}$$

Shift your perspective on challenges, initiating a quantum leap in consciousness and navigating adversity with newfound clarity.

**Emotional Alchemy Reaction:**

$$\text{Negative Emotions} \xrightarrow{\text{Mindfulness}} \text{Emotional Alchemy}$$

Engage in mindfulness as the alchemical process, transmuting negative emotions into sources of strength through profound self-awareness.

**Molecular Resilience Activation:**

$$\text{Resilient Beliefs} \xrightarrow{\text{Spiritual Resilience}} \text{Molecular Resilience Activation}$$

Activate molecular resilience by nurturing resilient beliefs through a foundation of spiritual practices.

**Neuroplasticity of Hope:**

$$\text{Hopeful Thoughts} \xrightarrow{\text{Spiritual Connection}} \text{Neuroplasticity Rewiring}$$

Rewire neural pathways with the neuroplasticity of hope, connecting to spirituality as a potent force for mental and emotional resilience.

**Holistic Healing Reaction:**

$$\text{Suffering} \xrightarrow{\text{Spiritual Alignment}} \text{Holistic Healing}$$

Initiate holistic healing by aligning with your spiritual essence, transcending suffering through a harmonious connection with the divine.

**Quantum Grace Dynamics:**

$$\text{Graceful Acceptance} \xleftrightarrow{\text{Spiritual Surrender}} \text{Quantum Resilience}$$

Achieve quantum resilience through the reciprocal dance of graceful acceptance and spiritual surrender.

**Psychological Equilibrium Equation:**

$$\text{Adversity Impact} \xrightarrow{\text{Spiritual Equilibrium}} \text{Psychological Stability}$$

Attain psychological stability by establishing spiritual equilibrium, minimizing the impact of adversity on your mental well-being.

**Transcendental Equation of Fortitude:**

$$\text{Spiritual Practices} \xrightarrow{\text{Inner Strength}} \text{Transcendental Fortitude}$$

Cultivate inner strength through dedicated spiritual practices, achieving a transcendental fortitude that empowers you to face any adversity.

Navigate life's challenges with grace and resilience, drawing strength from the wellspring of your spirituality.

# Chapter 12

# Therapeutic Arts and Creativity

## 12.1  Expressive Arts Therapy

Unleash the healing power of creativity through Expressive Arts Therapy.

**Creative Transformation Equation:**

$$\text{Inner Turmoil} \xrightarrow{\text{Expressive Arts}} \text{Creative Transformation}$$

Transform inner turmoil into a masterpiece of healing through the expressive arts, transcending pain with each stroke.

**Artistic Alchemy Reaction:**

$$\text{Emotional Chaos} \xrightarrow{\text{Artistic Expression}} \text{Artistic Alchemy}$$

Transmute emotional chaos into an artistic alchemy, where the canvas becomes a catalyst for emotional catharsis.

**Cathartic Release Formula:**

$$\text{Suppressed Feelings} \xrightarrow{\text{Creative Outlet}} \text{Cathartic Release}$$

Release suppressed feelings through creative outlets, discovering a therapeutic avenue for emotional catharsis.

**Sculpting Emotions Equation:**

$$\text{Raw Emotions} \xrightarrow{\text{Sculpting}} \text{Emotional Resilience}$$

Sculpt raw emotions into emotional resilience, molding the clay of experience into a form of strength and understanding.

**Visual Poetry Dynamics:**

$$\text{Silent Pain} \xrightarrow{\text{Visual Poetry}} \text{Expressive Liberation}$$

Translate silent pain into visual poetry, experiencing an expressive liberation that transcends the boundaries of spoken language.

**Creative Flow Reaction:**

$$\text{Stagnant Energy} \xrightarrow{\text{Creative Flow}} \text{Energy Renewal}$$

Revitalize stagnant energy through the creative flow, experiencing a renewal that sparks vitality and passion.

**Mindful Creation Formula:**

$$\text{Anxious Thoughts} \xrightarrow{\text{Mindful Creation}} \text{Calm Creations}$$

Channel anxious thoughts into mindful creation, witnessing the transformation of turmoil into serene and calming artworks.

**Artistic Therapeutic Resonance:**

$$\text{Artistic Expression} \xleftrightarrow{\text{Emotional Resonance}} \text{Therapeutic Harmony}$$

Establish a harmonious resonance between artistic expression and emotional well-being, creating therapeutic harmony.

**Creative Synthesis Dynamics:**

$$\text{Fragmented Emotions} \xrightarrow{\text{Creative Synthesis}} \text{Unified Expression}$$

Synthesize fragmented emotions through creative expression, achieving a unified and cohesive representation of the self.

**Colorful Healing Reaction:**

$$\text{Psychological Pain} \xrightarrow{\text{Colorful Expression}} \text{Healing Palette}$$

Paint a healing palette with colorful expression, transforming psychological pain into a work of art that soothes the soul.

**Holistic Artistry Equation:**

$$\text{Mind-Body Disharmony} \xrightarrow{\text{Holistic Artistry}} \text{Integrated Wellness}$$

Harmonize mind and body disharmony through holistic artistry, paving the way for integrated wellness and holistic healing.

Embark on a journey of self-discovery and healing through the transformative power of expressive arts therapy.

## 12.2  Writing as a Healing Tool

Unlock the healing potential of words through writing as a therapeutic tool.

**Ink of Resilience Formula:**

$$\text{Emotional Turmoil} \xrightarrow{\text{Writing}} \text{Ink of Resilience}$$

Transform emotional turmoil into the ink of resilience, where the written word becomes a powerful tool for inner strength.

**Narrative Empowerment Equation:**

$$\text{Personal Challenges} \xrightarrow{\text{Narrative Writing}} \text{Empowerment Story}$$

Confront personal challenges through narrative writing, crafting an empowerment story that reshapes the narrative of one's life.

**Therapeutic Reflection Reaction:**

$$\text{Life Confusion} \xrightarrow{\text{Reflective Writing}} \text{Therapeutic Clarity}$$

Navigate life's confusion with therapeutic reflection, gaining clarity through the written exploration of thoughts and feelings.

**Journaling Resurgence Formula:**

$$\text{Stagnant Emotions} \xrightarrow{\text{Journaling}} \text{Emotional Resurgence}$$

Revive stagnant emotions with journaling, experiencing an emotional resurgence that revitalizes the spirit.

**Expressive Language Dynamics:**

$$\text{Unspoken Grief} \xrightarrow{\text{Expressive Language}} \text{Verbal Liberation}$$

Give voice to unspoken grief through expressive language, achieving a verbal liberation that breaks the chains of silence.

**Poetic Catharsis Equation:**

$$\text{Heartache} \xrightarrow{\text{Poetry}} \text{Cathartic Verses}$$

Turn heartache into poetic catharsis, expressing emotions through verses that provide a profound release.

**Creative Writing Alchemy:**

$$\text{Creative Exploration} \xleftrightarrow{\text{Writing Alchemy}} \text{Therapeutic Transformation}$$

Engage in creative exploration and writing alchemy, creating a dynamic interplay that fosters therapeutic transformation.

**Storytelling Resilience Reaction:**

$$\text{Life Setbacks} \xrightarrow{\text{Storytelling}} \text{Resilient Narratives}$$

Navigate life setbacks through storytelling, shaping resilient narratives that become a source of strength.

**Symbolic Scripting Formula:**

$$\text{Inner Struggles} \xrightarrow{\text{Symbolic Writing}} \text{Scripted Empowerment}$$

Confront inner struggles through symbolic writing, scripting a narrative of empowerment that transcends challenges.

**Reflective Prose Dynamics:**

$$\text{Identity Exploration} \xrightarrow{\text{Reflective Prose}} \text{Self-Discovery Odyssey}$$

Embark on an identity exploration with reflective prose, uncovering a self-discovery odyssey through written reflection.

**Emotional Syntax Equation:**

$$\text{Chaos of Emotions} \xrightarrow{\text{Writing Syntax}} \text{Structured Serenity}$$

Bring order to the chaos of emotions with writing syntax, creating a structured serenity through the arrangement of words.

**Mindful Scripting Reaction:**

$$\text{Anxiety} \xrightarrow{\text{Mindful Writing}} \text{Calm Script}$$

Transform anxiety through mindful writing, crafting a calm script that promotes emotional well-being.

**Word Therapy Dynamics:**

$$\text{Emotional Distress} \xrightarrow{\text{Word Therapy}} \text{Healing Lexicon}$$

Heal emotional distress through word therapy, curating a healing lexicon that transforms pain into resilience.

Empower yourself with the written word, embracing writing as a therapeutic tool for healing and self-discovery.

## 12.3 Visual Arts for Emotional Expression

Unleash the power of emotions through visual arts as a tool for expression.

**Palette of Emotions Spectrum:**

$$\text{Inner Turmoil} \xrightarrow{\text{Visual Arts}} \text{Emotional Palette}$$

Translate inner turmoil into a spectrum of emotions using visual arts, creating an emotional palette that mirrors the soul.

**Colorful Catharsis Equation:**

$$\text{Emotional Distress} \xrightarrow{\text{Colorful Expression}} \text{Cathartic Release}$$

Express emotional distress through colorful art, experiencing a cathartic release that frees the spirit.

**Brushstroke Therapy Dynamics:**

$$\text{Anxiety} \xrightarrow{\text{Brushstrokes}} \text{Therapeutic Canvas}$$

Transform anxiety with each brushstroke, turning a canvas into a therapeutic space for emotional exploration.

**Sculpting Resilience Reaction:**

$$\text{Life Challenges} \xrightarrow{\text{Sculpting}} \text{Resilient Forms}$$

Mold life challenges into resilient forms through sculpting, shaping emotions into tangible expressions of strength.

**Visual Journaling Equation:**

$$\text{Daily Experiences} \xrightarrow{\text{Visual Journaling}} \text{Illustrated Narratives}$$

Capture daily experiences through visual journaling, crafting illustrated narratives that tell the story of one's journey.

**Photography Healing Reaction:**

$$\text{Painful Memories} \xrightarrow{\text{Photography}} \text{Healing Snapshots}$$

Heal from painful memories through photography, capturing snapshots that transform the past into healing art.

**Mixed Media Alchemy Formula:**

$$\text{Complex Emotions} \xleftrightarrow{\text{Mixed Media}} \text{Artistic Alchemy}$$

Engage with complex emotions through mixed media, creating an artistic alchemy that transforms the intangible into tangible beauty.

**Kinetic Emotion Reaction:**

$$\text{Restless Energy} \xrightarrow{\text{Kinetic Art}} \text{Emotion in Motion}$$

Channel restless energy into kinetic art, experiencing emotions in motion through dynamic visual expressions.

**Symbolic Art Equation:**

$$\text{Unspoken Feelings} \xrightarrow{\text{Symbolic Art}} \text{Artistic Language}$$

Convey unspoken feelings through symbolic art, creating an artistic language that communicates the inexpressible.

**Digital Art Therapy Dynamics:**

$$\text{Digital Expression} \xrightarrow{\text{Digital Art}} \text{Therapeutic Pixels}$$

Explore digital expression with digital art, transforming pixels into a therapeutic space for emotional processing.

**Artistic Reflection Reaction:**

$$\text{Self-Discovery} \xrightarrow{\text{Artistic Reflection}} \text{Mirror of Expression}$$

Embark on self-discovery through artistic reflection, using art as a mirror to express the depths of one's being.

**Artistic Mindfulness Equation:**

$$\text{Present Moment} \xrightarrow{\text{Artistic Mindfulness}} \text{Visual Serenity}$$

Attune to the present moment through artistic mindfulness, creating visual serenity through mindful artistic expressions.

**Art as Affirmation Dynamics:**

$$\text{Positive Affirmations} \xrightarrow{\text{Affirmative Art}} \text{Visual Manifestation}$$

Transform positive affirmations into visual manifestations through affirmative art, turning words into vibrant visuals.

Empower yourself through the visual language of art, utilizing it as a dynamic tool for emotional expression and self-discovery.

# 12.4 Music and Mood Regulation

Harmony in Sound Equation:

$$\text{Emotional Chaos} \xrightarrow{\text{Music}} \text{Harmonic Balance}$$

Immerse in the harmony of sound to transform emotional chaos into a state of harmonic balance. Rhythmic Resonance Formula:

$$\text{Dissonant Feelings} \xrightarrow{\text{Rhythm}} \text{Resonant Emotions}$$

Let the rhythm resonate with dissonant feelings, orchestrating a symphony of resonant emotions. Melodic Upliftment Reaction:

$$\text{Low Spirits} \xrightarrow{\text{Melody}} \text{Uplifted Soul}$$

Lift low spirits with a melodic embrace, elevating the soul through the power of musical notes.

Tempo of Tranquility Equation:

$$\text{Stress Intensity} \xrightarrow{\text{Calming Tempo}} \text{Tranquil State}$$

Adjust the tempo to a calming rhythm, reducing stress intensity and inducing a tranquil state.
Lyrically Guided Emotions:

$$\text{Conflicted Feelings} \xleftrightarrow{\text{Lyrics}} \text{Emotional Navigation}$$

Engage in lyrically guided emotions, allowing lyrics to navigate and express conflicted feelings.
Sonic Serenity Dynamics:

$$\text{Inner Turmoil} \xrightarrow{\text{Sonic Waves}} \text{Calm Waters}$$

Surf sonic waves to calm inner turmoil, turning the mental landscape into serene waters.
Chord Progression Therapy:

$$\text{Anxiety} \xrightarrow{\text{Chord Progression}} \text{Cathartic Harmony}$$

Undergo chord progression therapy, turning anxiety into a cathartic harmony of emotional release.
Musical Mindfulness Reaction:

$$\text{Overwhelmed Mind} \xrightarrow{\text{Musical Mindfulness}} \text{Present Harmony}$$

Practice musical mindfulness to shift from an overwhelmed mind to the present harmony of the
moment.
Harmonic Expression Formula:

$$\text{Suppressed Emotions} \xrightarrow{\text{Instrumental Expression}} \text{Harmonic Release}$$

Express suppressed emotions through instrumental means, achieving a harmonic release of pent-
up feelings.
Synchronized Sound Dynamics:

$$\text{Disconnected Emotions} \xleftrightarrow{\text{Synchronized Sound}} \text{Emotional Alignment}$$

Sync emotions with the power of sound, creating emotional alignment within the self.
Melancholy to Majestic Transformation:

$$\text{Melancholic State} \xrightarrow{\text{Orchestration}} \text{Majestic Elevation}$$

Transform a melancholic state through orchestration, reaching a majestic elevation of emotional experience.

Beat of Resilience Reaction:

$$\text{Setbacks and Struggles} \xrightarrow{\text{Beat Resilience}} \text{Rhythmic Resilience}$$

Build rhythmic resilience, using the beat to overcome setbacks and dance through life's struggles.

Musical Catharsis Equation:

$$\text{Emotional Burden} \xrightarrow{\text{Musical Release}} \text{Cathartic Liberation}$$

Release emotional burdens through musical expression, experiencing a cathartic liberation of the spirit.

Soulful Harmonization Dynamics:

$$\text{Internal Disharmony} \xleftrightarrow{\text{Soulful Harmony}} \text{Unified Self}$$

Attain a unified self by harmonizing internal disharmony through the soulful resonance of music.

Elevate your mood, regulate emotions, and find solace in the transformative power of music.

## 12.5  Dance and Movement Therapy

Kinetic Expression Dynamics:

$$\text{Internal Tension} \xrightarrow{\text{Movement}} \text{Expressive Liberation}$$

Release internal tension through movement, achieving expressive liberation and freeing the body and mind.

Rhythmic Resilience Equation:

$$\text{Life Challenges} \xrightarrow{\text{Dance}} \text{Resilient Adaptation}$$

Face life's challenges with dance, fostering rhythmic resilience and adapting with grace and strength.

Body-Mind Synchronization Formula:

$$\text{Cognitive Strain} \xleftrightarrow{\text{Synchronized Dance}} \text{Harmonized State}$$

Sync mind and body through dance, creating a harmonized state and alleviating cognitive strain.

Choreographic Catharsis Reaction:

$$\text{Emotional Blockages} \xrightarrow{\text{Choreography}} \text{Cathartic Expression}$$

Choreograph movements to break emotional blockages, allowing for cathartic expression and release.

Dance of Self-Discovery:

$$\text{Personal Exploration} \xrightarrow{\text{Dance Movements}} \text{Self-Understanding}$$

Embark on a dance of self-discovery, using movements to navigate and deepen self-understanding.

Balance in Ballet Equation:

$$\text{Life Imbalance} \xrightarrow{\text{Ballet}} \text{Equilibrium Achievement}$$

Achieve life balance through ballet, finding equilibrium and grace in the dance of existence.

Emotional Elevation Dynamics:

$$\text{Low Spirits} \xrightarrow{\text{Expressive Dance}} \text{Emotional Soaring}$$

Lift low spirits through expressive dance, soaring emotionally and finding joy in movement.

Dance of Empathy Formula:

$$\text{Empathy Deficit} \xleftrightarrow{\text{Partner Dance}} \text{Mutual Understanding}$$

Engage in partner dance for mutual understanding, bridging empathy deficits through shared movement.

Stress-Relief Salsa Reaction:

$$\text{Stress Accumulation} \xrightarrow{\text{Salsa}} \text{Stress Dissipation}$$

Dissipate accumulated stress with salsa, moving rhythmically to unwind and find stress relief.

Dance-Based Mindfulness Equation:

$$\text{Mind-Wandering} \xrightarrow{\text{Mindful Dance}} \text{Present-Moment Focus}$$

Combat mind-wandering through mindful dance, anchoring the mind in the present moment with each step.

Flow State Waltz Dynamics:

$$\text{Creativity Block} \xrightarrow{\text{Waltz}} \text{Creative Flow}$$

Break through creativity blocks with the waltz, entering a state of fluid and inspired creative flow.

Dance of Liberation Reaction:

$$\text{Feeling Restricted} \xrightarrow{\text{Freeform Dance}} \text{Liberated Spirit}$$

Liberate the spirit through freeform dance, breaking free from constraints and embracing movement.

Cultural Connection Tango:

$$\text{Cultural Disconnection} \xleftrightarrow{\text{Tango}} \text{Global Unity}$$

Connect cultures through the tango, fostering unity and understanding through the universal language of movement.

Therapeutic Tango Equation:

$$\text{Emotional Disconnection} \xrightarrow{\text{Tango Steps}} \text{Emotional Reconnection}$$

Reconnect emotionally through tango steps, using the dance to restore and strengthen emotional bonds.

Embodied Healing Dynamics:

$$\text{Physical Pain} \xrightarrow{\text{Healing Dance}} \text{Physical Well-being}$$

Heal physical pain through therapeutic dance, promoting physical well-being and holistic health.

Dance and movement therapy offer a profound path to physical, emotional, and mental well-being.

## 12.6 Incorporating Creativity into Daily Life

Creative Energy Activation:

$$\text{Routine Life} \xrightarrow{\text{Creativity}} \text{Energetic Vibrancy}$$

Inject creativity into routine life to activate a surge of energetic vibrancy, transforming the mundane into the extraordinary.

Daily Dose of Imagination Formula:

$$\text{Monotony} \xrightarrow{\text{Imaginative Sparks}} \text{Daily Adventure}$$

Infuse daily life with imaginative sparks to turn monotony into a daily adventure, exploring new realms of possibility.

Artistic Breakthrough Reaction:

$$\text{Stagnation} \xrightarrow{\text{Creative Breakthrough}} \text{Artistic Renewal}$$

Break through stagnation with creative impulses, experiencing an artistic renewal of mind and spirit.

Innovative Problem-Solving Equation:

$$\text{Challenges} \xrightarrow{\text{Creative Solutions}} \text{Innovative Triumph}$$

Confront challenges with creative solutions, turning obstacles into stepping stones toward innovative triumph.

Spontaneity Unleashed Reaction:

$$\text{Predictability} \xrightarrow{\text{Spontaneous Moments}} \text{Unleashed Joy}$$

Shatter predictability with spontaneous moments, unleashing waves of joy and embracing the unexpected.

Doodle Therapy Dynamics:

$$\text{Stressful Thoughts} \xrightarrow{\text{Doodling}} \text{Visual Serenity}$$

Channel stressful thoughts into doodling, creating visual serenity and a therapeutic escape from mental tension.

Creative Mindfulness Reaction:

$$\text{Overthinking} \xrightarrow{\text{Creative Focus}} \text{Mindful Presence}$$

Shift from overthinking to creative focus, cultivating mindful presence in the current moment.

Inspirational Environment Formula:

$$\text{Bland Surroundings} \xrightarrow{\text{Creative Decor}} \text{Inspired Spaces}$$

Transform bland surroundings with creative decor, turning spaces into inspirational havens that spark imagination.

Expressive Journaling Dynamics:

$$\text{Silent Reflection} \xrightarrow{\text{Expressive Journaling}} \text{Emotional Release}$$

Use expressive journaling for silent reflection, facilitating emotional release and fostering self-discovery.

Crafting Connection Equation:

$$\text{Isolation} \xrightarrow{\text{Creative Gatherings}} \text{Community Bonds}$$

Combat isolation with creative gatherings, weaving community bonds through shared artistic expression.

Mindful Crafting Reaction:

$$\text{Restlessness} \xrightarrow{\text{Crafting}} \text{Calm Creations}$$

Transform restlessness into calm creations through the mindful process of crafting.

Creativity as a Coping Mechanism:

$$\text{Adversity} \xrightarrow{\text{Creative Coping}} \text{Resilient Spirit}$$

Employ creativity as a coping mechanism during adversity, nurturing a resilient spirit and adaptive mindset.

Artistic Rituals Formula:

$$\text{Daily Routine} \xrightarrow{\text{Artistic Rituals}} \text{Daily Celebrations}$$

Infuse daily routines with artistic rituals, turning ordinary moments into daily celebrations of creativity.

Playful Imagination Dynamics:

$$\text{Serious Atmosphere} \xrightarrow{\text{Playful Imagination}} \text{Lighter Perspectives}$$

Introduce playful imagination to a serious atmosphere, inviting lighter perspectives and a more joyful outlook.

Unlock the power of creativity in daily life, turning every moment into an opportunity for imaginative expression.

## 12.7 The Therapeutic Power of Nature

Natural Healing Equation:

$$\text{Stress} \xrightarrow{\text{Nature Exposure}} \text{Calming Relief}$$

Combat stress by immersing yourself in nature, experiencing the therapeutic equation that brings calming relief.

Sunlight Therapy Dynamics:

$$\text{Low Energy} \xrightarrow{\text{Sunlight Exposure}} \text{Vitality Boost}$$

Revitalize low energy levels with sunlight exposure, providing a natural boost to vitality.

Forest Bathing Reaction:

$$\text{Mental Fatigue} \xrightarrow{\text{Forest Bathing}} \text{Cognitive Refreshment}$$

Overcome mental fatigue through forest bathing, fostering cognitive refreshment in the embrace of nature.

Nature's Breathing Formula:

$$\text{Anxiety} \xrightarrow{\text{Deep Nature Breaths}} \text{Tranquil Mindset}$$

Alleviate anxiety with deep nature breaths, cultivating a tranquil mindset through the rhythm of the natural world.

Floral Aromatherapy Reaction:

$$\text{Tension} \xrightarrow{\text{Floral Scents}} \text{Relaxed State}$$

Release tension with floral scents, inducing a relaxed state through the therapeutic power of aromatherapy.

Biophilic Design Equation:

$$\text{Indoor Stress} \xrightarrow{\text{Biophilic Spaces}} \text{Balanced Well-being}$$

Counter indoor stress with biophilic design, creating balanced well-being through connections with nature indoors.

Eco-Therapeutic Meditation Dynamics:

$$\text{Restless Thoughts} \xrightarrow{\text{Eco-Meditation}} \text{Mindful Serenity}$$

Calm restless thoughts through eco-therapeutic meditation, achieving mindful serenity with nature as a guide.

Green Exercise Reaction:

$$\text{Physical Inactivity} \xrightarrow{\text{Green Workouts}} \text{Physical and Mental Fitness}$$

Combat physical inactivity with green workouts, promoting both physical and mental fitness through outdoor activities.

Natural Symmetry Equation:

$$\text{Chaos} \xrightarrow{\text{Nature's Symmetry}} \text{Harmony Restoration}$$

Restore harmony in the face of chaos by observing nature's symmetry, finding balance in the patterns of the natural world.

Aquatic Mindfulness Reaction:

$$\text{Stagnant Thoughts} \xrightarrow{\text{Water Contemplation}} \text{Flowing Clarity}$$

Clear stagnant thoughts with water contemplation, attaining flowing clarity through mindful connection with aquatic environments.

Birdsong Therapy Formula:

$$\text{Noise Pollution} \xrightarrow{\text{Birdsong Melodies}} \text{Auditory Comfort}$$

Escape noise pollution with birdsong melodies, finding auditory comfort in the soothing sounds of nature.

Nature-Inspired Creativity Reaction:

$$\text{Creative Block} \xrightarrow{\text{Nature-Inspired Art}} \text{Artistic Flow}$$

Break creative blocks by engaging in nature-inspired art, unlocking an artistic flow inspired by the beauty of the natural world.

Biodiversity Wellness Equation:

$$\text{Monotonous Environment} \xrightarrow{\text{Biodiverse Spaces}} \text{Mental Stimulation}$$

Transform a monotonous environment into biodiverse spaces, providing mental stimulation through encounters with diverse ecosystems.

Quantum Nature Connection:

$$\text{Disconnect} \xrightarrow{\text{Quantum Nature Bond}} \text{Connected Consciousness}$$

Reconnect with nature to overcome feelings of disconnect, fostering a quantum nature bond for a connected consciousness.

Tap into the therapeutic power of nature, allowing it to be your guide on a journey to holistic well-being.

# Chapter 13

# Mind-Body Techniques

## 13.1 Biofeedback and Stress Reduction

Stress Reduction Formula:

$$\text{Stress} \xrightarrow{\text{Biofeedback Techniques}} \text{Calmness}$$

Harness the power of biofeedback techniques to transform stress into a state of calmness, achieving mental tranquility.

Heart Coherence Equation:

$$\text{Irregular Heartbeat} \xrightarrow{\text{Biofeedback Training}} \text{Heart Coherence}$$

Train the heart with biofeedback to shift from irregular beats to heart coherence, promoting cardiovascular well-being.

Breath Awareness Reaction:

$$\text{Shallow Breathing} \xrightarrow{\text{Biofeedback Monitoring}} \text{Deep Respiratory Harmony}$$

Monitor breathing with biofeedback to transition from shallow breaths to deep respiratory harmony, fostering relaxation.

Muscle Tension Release Formula:

$$\text{Tense Muscles} \xrightarrow{\text{Biofeedback Sensors}} \text{Muscle Relaxation}$$

Utilize biofeedback sensors to detect tense muscles and initiate a response for muscle relaxation, relieving physical tension.

Galvanic Skin Response Dynamics:

$$\text{Stressful Situations} \xrightarrow{\text{Biofeedback}} \text{Galvanic Skin Stability}$$

Apply biofeedback in stressful situations to achieve galvanic skin stability, indicating a balanced physiological response.

Temperature Biofeedback Equation:

$$\text{Temperature Variations} \xrightarrow{\text{Biofeedback Training}} \text{Thermal Self-Regulation}$$

Engage in biofeedback training to regulate temperature variations, fostering thermal self-regulation for stress relief.

Brainwave Synchronization Reaction:

$$\text{Mind Racing} \xrightarrow{\text{Neurofeedback}} \text{Cognitive Harmony}$$

Employ neurofeedback techniques to synchronize brainwaves, transitioning from a racing mind to cognitive harmony.

Electromyography (EMG) Therapy:

$$\text{Muscle Tension} \xrightarrow{\text{EMG Biofeedback}} \text{Muscular Relaxation}$$

Integrate EMG biofeedback to address muscle tension, promoting muscular relaxation and overall well-being.

Heart Rate Variability (HRV) Formula:

$$\text{Inconsistent Heart Rate} \xrightarrow{\text{HRV Biofeedback}} \text{Heart Rate Coherence}$$

Engage in HRV biofeedback to transform inconsistent heart rate into heart rate coherence, enhancing cardiovascular health.

Cognitive Focus Dynamics:

$$\text{Mind Distractions} \xrightarrow{\text{Biofeedback Techniques}} \text{Concentration Mastery}$$

Apply biofeedback techniques to conquer mind distractions, achieving mastery in concentration and mental focus.

Visual Biofeedback Reaction:

$$\text{Stressful Imagery} \xrightarrow{\text{Visual Feedback}} \text{Relaxing Mental Imagery}$$

Utilize visual biofeedback to alter stressful mental imagery, replacing it with relaxing and calming mental pictures.

Mind-Body Connection Equation:

$$\text{Disconnected State} \xrightarrow{\text{Biofeedback Integration}} \text{Holistic Well-Being}$$

Integrate biofeedback techniques for a seamless mind-body connection, promoting holistic well-being and balance.

Biofeedback tools empower you to take control, promoting a harmonious mind-body relationship for stress reduction and improved mental health.

## 13.2  Guided Imagery for Relaxation

Imagery Impact Formula:

$$\text{Stressful Thoughts} \xrightarrow{\text{Guided Imagery}} \text{Calming Mental Images}$$

Transform stressful thoughts using guided imagery into calming mental images, fostering relaxation and tranquility.

Mind's Eye Visualization:

$$\text{Overwhelm} \xrightarrow{\text{Guided Imagery Techniques}} \text{Calm Mind's Eye}$$

Utilize guided imagery techniques to transition from overwhelm to a calm mind's eye visualization, promoting mental serenity.

Breath-Linked Imagery:

$$\text{Anxiety} \xrightarrow{\text{Guided Breath Imagery}} \text{Breath-Linked Calmness}$$

Incorporate guided breath imagery to associate anxiety with breath-linked calmness, promoting a soothing effect.

Nature Immersion Equation:

$$\text{Stressful Environment} \xrightarrow{\text{Guided Nature Imagery}} \text{Mental Oasis}$$

Engage in guided nature imagery to turn a stressful environment into a mental oasis, providing a mental escape.

Temporal Distortion Reaction:

$$\text{Time Pressure} \xrightarrow{\text{Guided Imagery}} \text{Time Expansion Perception}$$

Use guided imagery to alter time pressure perception, creating a sense of time expansion and reducing urgency.

Spatial Visualization Formula:

$$\text{Confined Space} \xrightarrow{\text{Guided Visualization}} \text{Expansive Mental Space}$$

Practice guided visualization to transform confined spaces into expansive mental landscapes, fostering a sense of freedom.

Color Therapy Dynamics:

$$\text{Mental Turbulence} \xrightarrow{\text{Guided Imagery with Colors}} \text{Color-Infused Calmness}$$

Apply guided imagery with colors to alleviate mental turbulence, infusing calmness through the power of color therapy.

Sensory Imagery Reaction:

$$\text{Stressful Situations} \xrightarrow{\text{Multi-Sensory Imagery}} \text{Sensory Harmony}$$

Engage in multi-sensory guided imagery to harmonize the senses during stressful situations, promoting overall well-being.

Healing Visualization Equation:

$$\text{Pain or Discomfort} \xrightarrow{\text{Guided Healing Imagery}} \text{Pain Alleviation Perception}$$

Practice guided healing imagery to shift the perception of pain or discomfort, contributing to pain alleviation.

Emotional Reservoir Dynamics:

$$\text{Emotional Drain} \xrightarrow{\text{Guided Imagery Techniques}} \text{Emotional Reservoir Replenishment}$$

Use guided imagery techniques to replenish the emotional reservoir, restoring emotional balance and stability.

Future Self Visualization:

$$\text{Uncertainty} \xrightarrow{\text{Guided Imagery}} \text{Confident Future-Self Image}$$

Combat uncertainty through guided imagery by envisioning a confident future-self image, fostering resilience and optimism.

Guided imagery offers a powerful mental toolset, transforming stressful thoughts into tranquil mental landscapes for enhanced relaxation and well-being.

## 13.3　Progressive Muscle Relaxation

Relaxation Response Equation:

$$\text{Tense Muscles} \xrightarrow{\text{PMR Technique}} \text{Muscular Relaxation}$$

Master the Progressive Muscle Relaxation (PMR) technique to shift from tense muscles to deep muscular relaxation, fostering tranquility.

Tension Release Formula:

$$\text{Muscle Contraction} \xrightarrow{\text{PMR}} \text{Muscle Release}$$

Engage in PMR to release muscle contractions systematically, promoting muscle release and overall physical comfort.

Deep Breathing Synchronization:

$$\text{Shallow Breaths} \xrightarrow{\text{Combined with PMR}} \text{Deep Respiratory Harmony}$$

Combine PMR with deep breathing for a synchronized approach, transitioning from shallow breaths to deep respiratory harmony.

Stress-Relief Dynamics:

$$\text{Stressful Situations} \xrightarrow{\text{PMR Practice}} \text{Calmness}$$

Incorporate PMR into your routine to counteract stress in various situations, promoting a consistent state of calmness.

Cognitive Relaxation Equation:

$$\text{Anxious Thoughts} \xrightarrow{\text{PMR Techniques}} \text{Cognitive Serenity}$$

Apply PMR techniques to alleviate anxious thoughts, achieving cognitive serenity and mental tranquility.

Sleep Quality Improvement:

$$\text{Restlessness} \xrightarrow{\text{PMR Before Sleep}} \text{Quality Sleep}$$

Practice PMR before sleep to transform restlessness into quality sleep, enhancing overall sleep duration and efficiency.

Body-Mind Harmony Reaction:

$$\text{Body Tension} \xrightarrow{\text{PMR Integration}} \text{Holistic Well-Being}$$

Integrate PMR into your lifestyle for a harmonious body-mind connection, contributing to holistic well-being.

Neuromuscular Calmness Formula:

$$\text{Neuromuscular Activation} \xrightarrow{\text{PMR Practices}} \text{Neuromuscular Calmness}$$

Incorporate PMR practices to induce neuromuscular calmness, promoting a balanced and relaxed state of being.

Physical and Mental Equilibrium:

$$\text{Physical Strain} \xrightarrow{\text{PMR Routine}} \text{Mental-Energetic Balance}$$

Establish a regular PMR routine to counter physical strain, cultivating a state of mental-energetic balance.

Mindful Relaxation Reaction:

$$\text{Mind-Wandering} \xrightarrow{\text{PMR Focus}} \text{Mindful Relaxation}$$

Channel your focus with PMR techniques to shift from mind-wandering to a state of mindful relaxation.

Emotional Release Equation:

$$\text{Emotional Tension} \xrightarrow{\text{Combined with PMR}} \text{Emotional Release}$$

Combine PMR with emotional awareness for a dual approach, facilitating both physical and emotional tension release.

Positive Affirmation Integration:

$$\text{Negative Energy} \xrightarrow{\text{PMR Affirmations}} \text{Positive Mindset}$$

Incorporate positive affirmations during PMR for a transformative experience, turning negative energy into a positive mindset.

Progressive Muscle Relaxation is your gateway to a more relaxed, comfortable, and harmonious physical and mental state. Practice regularly for optimal well-being.

## 13.4 Breathwork for Mental Well-being

### 13.4.1 Breathing Equilibrium Formula:

$$\text{Irregular Breathing} \xrightarrow{\text{Breathwork Techniques}} \text{Respiratory Equilibrium}$$

Adopt specialized breathwork techniques to transform irregular breathing patterns into a state of respiratory equilibrium, promoting mental well-being.

### 13.4.2 Oxygenation Dynamics:

$$\text{Shallow Breaths} \xrightarrow{\text{Deep Breath Exercises}} \text{Optimal Oxygenation}$$

Engage in deep breath exercises to transition from shallow breaths to optimal oxygenation, enhancing overall cognitive function and mental clarity.

### 13.4.3 Stress Dissipation Reaction:

$$\text{Stressful Situations} \xrightarrow{\text{Mindful Breathing}} \text{Calmness}$$

Practice mindful breathing in stressful situations to dissipate stress, fostering a sense of calmness and mental resilience.

### 13.4.4 $CO_2$ Regulation Formula:

$$CO_2 \text{ Imbalance} \xrightarrow{\text{Breath Control}} CO_2 \text{ Homeostasis}$$

Implement breath control techniques to restore $CO_2$ balance, contributing to $CO_2$ homeostasis and mental stability.

### 13.4.5   Brain Oxygen Infusion:

$$\text{Oxygen Deficiency} \xrightarrow{\text{Conscious Breathing}} \text{Brain Oxygenation}$$

Consciously regulate breathing to counteract oxygen deficiency, infusing the brain with optimal oxygen levels for heightened mental function.

### 13.4.6   Cognitive Reset Reaction:

$$\text{Overthinking} \xrightarrow{\text{Focused Breathing}} \text{Cognitive Reset}$$

Apply focused breathing to interrupt overthinking patterns, facilitating a cognitive reset and promoting mental clarity.

### 13.4.7   Emotional Resilience Equation:

$$\text{Emotional Turbulence} \xrightarrow{\text{Breathwork Practices}} \text{Emotional Resilience}$$

Incorporate breathwork practices to navigate emotional turbulence, fostering emotional resilience and stability.

### 13.4.8   Heart Rate Variability (HRV) Optimization:

$$\text{Fluctuating HRV} \xrightarrow{\text{Breath Rhythm Regulation}} \text{Optimized HRV}$$

Regulate breath rhythm to optimize heart rate variability (HRV), creating a harmonious physiological state that positively influences mental well-being.

### 13.4.9   Sympathetic-Parasympathetic Balance:

$$\text{Sympathetic Dominance} \xrightarrow{\text{Balanced Breathing}} \text{Sympathetic-Parasympathetic Equilibrium}$$

Practice balanced breathing to shift from sympathetic dominance to a state of sympathetic-parasympathetic equilibrium, enhancing mental balance.

### 13.4.10   Mindful Breath Integration:

$$\text{Mind-Wandering} \xrightarrow{\text{Conscious Breathing}} \text{Mindful Presence}$$

Integrate conscious breathing into daily life to transition from mind-wandering to a state of mindful presence, promoting mental well-being.

Breathwork for mental well-being is a powerful tool for achieving a balanced and resilient mind. Incorporate these techniques into your routine for optimal mental health.

## 13.5 Yoga and Mindfulness Practices

### 13.5.1 Yoga Equilibrium Sequence:

$$\text{Physical Tension} \xrightarrow{\text{Yoga Poses}} \text{Mind-Body Equilibrium}$$

Engage in yoga poses to alleviate physical tension, fostering a state of mind-body equilibrium for enhanced well-being.

### 13.5.2 Mindful Movement Formula:

$$\text{Mindless Actions} \xrightarrow{\text{Mindful Yoga}} \text{Conscious Living}$$

Incorporate mindful yoga into daily activities to shift from mindless actions to conscious living, promoting mental presence and awareness.

### 13.5.3 Balance Asana Equation:

$$\text{Inner Imbalance} \xrightarrow{\text{Balancing Poses}} \text{Inner Harmony}$$

Practice balancing yoga poses to address inner imbalance, cultivating a sense of inner harmony and mental stability.

### 13.5.4 Breath-Body Synchronization:

$$\text{Disconnected Breath} \xrightarrow{\text{Yogic Breathing}} \text{Unified Breath-Body}$$

Utilize yogic breathing to synchronize breath and body, creating a unified state that positively influences mental and emotional well-being.

### 13.5.5 Mindful Posture Integration:

$$\text{Slouched Posture} \xrightarrow{\text{Conscious Alignment}} \text{Mindful Posture}$$

Consciously align the body during yoga for a mindful posture, positively impacting mental confidence and self-perception.

### 13.5.6  Yogic Relaxation Response:

$$\text{Stress Activation} \xrightarrow{\text{Savasana}} \text{Relaxation Mode}$$

Enter the relaxation mode through the Savasana pose to deactivate stress responses, promoting mental relaxation and rejuvenation.

### 13.5.7  Flow State Induction:

$$\text{Mental Stagnation} \xrightarrow{\text{Yoga Flow}} \text{Mental Flow State}$$

Immerse in yoga flow sequences to transition from mental stagnation to a state of mental flow, fostering creativity and focus.

### 13.5.8  Mindfulness Meditation Integration:

$$\text{Restless Mind} \xrightarrow{\text{Yoga Meditation}} \text{Mindful Tranquility}$$

Incorporate yoga meditation to calm a restless mind, cultivating mindful tranquility for improved mental clarity.

### 13.5.9  Chakra Balancing Formula:

$$\text{Energy Blockages} \xrightarrow{\text{Chakra-focused Poses}} \text{Energetic Balance}$$

Engage in poses that focus on specific chakras to release energy blockages, establishing energetic balance and mental vitality.

### 13.5.10  Yoga Nidra Relaxation:

$$\text{Sleep Disruptions} \xrightarrow{\text{Yoga Nidra}} \text{Restful Sleep}$$

Practice Yoga Nidra for deep relaxation to overcome sleep disruptions, ensuring restful sleep and supporting mental resilience.

Yoga and mindfulness practices are potent tools for cultivating a harmonious connection between the mind and body. Incorporate these techniques into your routine for optimal mental and physical well-being.

## 13.6 Tai Chi for Stress Reduction

### 13.6.1 Tai Chi Harmony Equation:

$$\text{Stressful State} \xrightarrow{\text{Tai Chi Movements}} \text{Inner Harmony}$$

Engage in Tai Chi movements to transform a stressful state into a state of inner harmony, promoting mental and emotional balance.

### 13.6.2 Mindful Motion Formula:

$$\text{Mind-wandering} \xrightarrow{\text{Tai Chi Focus}} \text{Mindful Presence}$$

Immerse in the focus of Tai Chi to shift from mind-wandering to mindful presence, fostering mental clarity and stress reduction.

### 13.6.3 Balance Flow Dynamics:

$$\text{Internal Imbalance} \xrightarrow{\text{Tai Chi Flow}} \text{Dynamic Equilibrium}$$

Practice Tai Chi's flowing movements to address internal imbalance, creating a dynamic equilibrium for enhanced mental well-being.

### 13.6.4 Breath-Movement Synchronization:

$$\text{Disrupted Breath} \xrightarrow{\text{Tai Chi Breathing}} \text{Harmonized Breath-Movement}$$

Incorporate Tai Chi breathing techniques to synchronize breath and movement, fostering a harmonized state for stress reduction.

### 13.6.5 Mindful Posture Alignment:

$$\text{Tense Posture} \xrightarrow{\text{Tai Chi Postures}} \text{Relaxed Posture}$$

Adopt Tai Chi postures for a shift from tense to relaxed posture, positively influencing mental relaxation and stress relief.

### 13.6.6   Tai Chi Stress Resilience:

$$\text{Stress Impact} \xrightarrow{\text{Tai Chi Practice}} \text{Stress Resilience}$$

Regular Tai Chi practice mitigates the impact of stress, enhancing stress resilience and supporting mental well-being.

### 13.6.7   Flowing Meditation State:

$$\text{Mental Turbulence} \xrightarrow{\text{Tai Chi Meditation}} \text{Calm Flow State}$$

Integrate Tai Chi meditation to calm mental turbulence, inducing a state of calm flow and stress reduction.

### 13.6.8   Energy Flow Optimization:

$$\text{Blocked Energy} \xrightarrow{\text{Tai Chi Energy Flow}} \text{Optimized Vitality}$$

Engage in Tai Chi to facilitate the flow of energy, unblocking stagnant energy for optimized vitality and reduced stress.

### 13.6.9   Tai Chi Mindful Relaxation:

$$\text{Restless Mindset} \xrightarrow{\text{Tai Chi Relaxation}} \text{Tranquil Mindset}$$

Utilize Tai Chi relaxation techniques to ease a restless mindset, cultivating a tranquil mental state and reducing stress.

### 13.6.10   Tai Chi Mind-Body Harmony:

$$\text{Stressful Tension} \xrightarrow{\text{Tai Chi Integration}} \text{Mind-Body Harmony}$$

Integrate Tai Chi into daily life to dissolve stressful tension, promoting a harmonious connection between the mind and body.

Tai Chi serves as a powerful practice for reducing stress and promoting mental well-being. Embrace these principles to enhance your mental resilience and cultivate a state of inner peace.

## 13.7 Holistic Approaches to Physical Health

### 13.7.1 Balanced Nutrition Equation:

$$\text{Nutrient Intake} \xrightarrow{\text{Holistic Diet}} \text{Body Harmony}$$

Adopt a holistic diet for optimal nutrient intake, fostering body harmony and supporting overall physical health.

### 13.7.2 Hydration Balance Formula:

$$\text{Dehydration} \xrightarrow{\text{Hydration Practices}} \text{Fluid Equilibrium}$$

Incorporate hydration practices to combat dehydration, maintaining fluid equilibrium for improved physical well-being.

### 13.7.3 Sleep Quality Optimization:

$$\text{Sleep Disruption} \xrightarrow{\text{Holistic Sleep Hygiene}} \text{Restful Sleep}$$

Prioritize holistic sleep hygiene to mitigate sleep disruption, ensuring restful sleep and promoting physical recovery.

### 13.7.4 Exercise for Vitality:

$$\text{Sedentary Lifestyle} \xrightarrow{\text{Holistic Exercise}} \text{Physical Vitality}$$

Embrace holistic exercise routines to counter a sedentary lifestyle, fostering physical vitality and overall health.

### 13.7.5 Stress-Relief Fitness:

$$\text{Stress Impact} \xrightarrow{\text{Holistic Fitness Practices}} \text{Stress Resilience}$$

Engage in holistic fitness practices to mitigate stress impact, enhancing stress resilience and supporting physical health.

### 13.7.6   Body-Mind Alignment:

$$\text{Physical Discomfort} \xrightarrow{\text{Holistic Practices}} \text{Mind-Body Harmony}$$

Incorporate holistic practices to alleviate physical discomfort, promoting mind-body harmony and overall well-being.

### 13.7.7   Holistic Body Detox:

$$\text{Toxic Buildup} \xrightarrow{\text{Detox Strategies}} \text{Purified System}$$

Implement holistic detox strategies to combat toxic buildup, ensuring a purified system for enhanced physical health.

### 13.7.8   Immune Support Equation:

$$\text{Immune Vulnerability} \xrightarrow{\text{Holistic Immune Support}} \text{Robust Immunity}$$

Prioritize holistic immune support to fortify immune defenses, fostering robust immunity and overall health.

### 13.7.9   Mindful Movement Practices:

$$\text{Physical Stagnation} \xrightarrow{\text{Holistic Movement}} \text{Energetic Flow}$$

Embrace holistic movement practices to counter physical stagnation, encouraging energetic flow and improved physical health.

### 13.7.10   Holistic Pain Management:

$$\text{Painful Sensations} \xrightarrow{\text{Comprehensive Approaches}} \text{Comfortable Living}$$

Apply comprehensive holistic approaches to manage painful sensations, promoting comfortable living and physical well-being.

Holistic approaches to physical health encompass a range of practices that synergistically contribute to overall well-being. Integrate these principles into your lifestyle for a healthier, more vibrant life.

# Chapter 14

# Thriving Beyond Depression

## 14.1 Embracing a Fulfilling Life

### 14.1.1 Vibrant Life Equation:

$$\text{Depression} \xrightarrow{\text{Holistic Lifestyle}} \text{Vibrant Living}$$

Overcome depression by adopting a holistic lifestyle, paving the way for vibrant living and overall well-being.

### 14.1.2 Passion Activation Formula:

$$\text{Lack of Interest} \xrightarrow{\text{Discovering Passions}} \text{Fulfillment}$$

Combat lack of interest through discovering passions, unlocking a path to fulfillment and joyous living.

### 14.1.3 Social Connection Algorithm:

$$\text{Isolation} \xrightarrow{\text{Social Engagement}} \text{Community Support}$$

Alleviate isolation by engaging socially, fostering community support and enhancing emotional resilience.

### 14.1.4 Mind-Body Rejuvenation:

$$\text{Mental Exhaustion} \xrightarrow{\text{Holistic Self-Care}} \text{Renewed Energy}$$

Combat mental exhaustion with holistic self-care, rejuvenating the mind and cultivating renewed energy.

### 14.1.5 Goal Achievement Dynamics:

$$\text{Lack of Direction} \xrightarrow{\text{Setting Achievable Goals}} \text{Empowerment}$$

Address a lack of direction through setting achievable goals, empowering yourself towards a purposeful life.

### 14.1.6 Gratitude Amplification:

$$\text{Negative Outlook} \xrightarrow{\text{Cultivating Gratitude}} \text{Positive Mindset}$$

Transform a negative outlook by cultivating gratitude, amplifying a positive mindset for mental well-being.

### 14.1.7 Nature Connection Algorithm:

$$\text{Indoor Confinement} \xrightarrow{\text{Outdoor Exploration}} \text{Natural Resilience}$$

Escape indoor confinement with outdoor exploration, nurturing a connection with nature for enhanced resilience.

### 14.1.8 Mindful Presence Equation:

$$\text{Ruminating Thoughts} \xrightarrow{\text{Mindfulness Practices}} \text{Present Serenity}$$

Overcome ruminating thoughts through mindfulness practices, attaining present serenity and mental peace.

### 14.1.9 Positive Affirmation Blueprint:

$$\text{Self-Doubt} \xrightarrow{\text{Affirmation Integration}} \text{Self-Confidence}$$

Combat self-doubt by integrating positive affirmations, fostering self-confidence and a resilient mindset.

### 14.1.10  Creative Expression Dynamics:

$$\text{Suppressed Emotions} \xrightarrow{\text{Artistic Outlets}} \text{Emotional Release}$$

Release suppressed emotions through artistic outlets, achieving emotional release and fostering catharsis.

Thriving beyond depression involves embracing a fulfilling life through holistic strategies. Incorporate these practices into your journey, unlocking the path to lasting well-being and fulfillment.

## 14.2  Contributing to Others

### 14.2.1  Generosity Quotient:

$$\text{Self-Focus} \xrightarrow{\text{Acts of Generosity}} \text{Community Impact}$$

Shift from self-focus by engaging in acts of generosity, creating a positive community impact and fostering a sense of purpose.

### 14.2.2  Social Altruism Formula:

$$\text{Isolation} \xrightarrow{\text{Social Contribution}} \text{Connection Resilience}$$

Combat isolation through social contribution, building connection resilience and forming meaningful relationships.

### 14.2.3  Empathy Amplification:

$$\text{Internal Struggle} \xrightarrow{\text{Empathetic Actions}} \text{Emotional Healing}$$

Address internal struggles with empathetic actions, contributing to emotional healing for oneself and others.

### 14.2.4  Collaborative Wellness Equation:

$$\text{Individual Healing} \xrightarrow{\text{Community Support}} \text{Collective Well-being}$$

Extend individual healing by participating in community support, contributing to collective well-being and shared resilience.

### 14.2.5   Impactful Service Dynamics:

$$\text{Sense of Insignificance} \xrightarrow{\text{Meaningful Service}} \text{Empowerment}$$

Overcome a sense of insignificance through meaningful service, empowering oneself and others towards positive change.

### 14.2.6   Time Investment Multiplier:

$$\text{Idle Moments} \xrightarrow{\text{Volunteer Commitment}} \text{Time Well-Spent}$$

Transform idle moments by committing to volunteer activities, multiplying time investment for a sense of purpose and fulfillment.

### 14.2.7   Positive Ripple Effect:

$$\text{Positive Actions} \xrightarrow{\text{Inspirational Influence}} \text{Widespread Positivity}$$

Engage in positive actions, creating an inspirational influence with a ripple effect, spreading positivity in the community.

### 14.2.8   Mindful Contribution Blueprint:

$$\text{Unfocused Energy} \xrightarrow{\text{Mindful Service}} \text{Calm Empowerment}$$

Channel unfocused energy through mindful service, cultivating calm empowerment for oneself and making a difference.

### 14.2.9   Building Support Networks:

$$\text{Limited Connections} \xrightarrow{\text{Supportive Communities}} \text{Unified Strength}$$

Address limited connections by joining supportive communities, building networks that contribute to unified strength.

### 14.2.10   Gratitude Reciprocity:

$$\text{Receiving Help} \xrightarrow{\text{Expressing Gratitude}} \text{Positive Loop}$$

Express gratitude when receiving help, creating a positive loop of reciprocal support and reinforcing a sense of community.

Contributing to others is a powerful avenue for thriving beyond depression. Embrace these strategies to not only make a positive impact on those around you but also to enhance your own well-being in the process.

## 14.3 Continued Growth and Development

### 14.3.1 Personal Evolution Equation:

$$\text{Current State} \xrightarrow{\text{Continuous Learning}} \text{Evolving Self}$$

Constantly engage in learning and self-improvement, fostering a journey of personal evolution and growth.

### 14.3.2 Resilience Building Formula:

$$\text{Past Challenges} \xrightarrow{\text{Adaptive Skills}} \text{Resilient Future}$$

Transform past challenges into opportunities for developing adaptive skills, ensuring a resilient approach to future endeavors.

### 14.3.3 Goal Achievement Dynamics:

$$\text{Aspirations} \xrightarrow{\text{Strategic Planning}} \text{Goal Attainment}$$

Translate aspirations into actionable plans, strategically navigating the path to achieve personal and professional goals.

### 14.3.4 Emotional Intelligence Blueprint:

$$\text{Emotional Awareness} \xrightarrow{\text{Emotion Regulation}} \text{Mental Fortitude}$$

Enhance emotional intelligence through awareness and regulation, cultivating mental fortitude for navigating life's ups and downs.

### 14.3.5 Continuous Skills Enhancement:

$$\text{Current Skills} \xrightarrow{\text{Skill Refinement}} \text{Competitive Edge}$$

Refine existing skills and acquire new ones, maintaining a competitive edge in personal and professional spheres.

### 14.3.6  Holistic Wellness Equation:

$$\text{Mind-Body Harmony} \xrightarrow{\text{Healthy Practices}} \text{Overall Well-being}$$

Foster mind-body harmony through healthy practices, contributing to overall well-being and sustained growth.

### 14.3.7  Positive Habit Formation:

$$\text{Behavioral Patterns} \xrightarrow{\text{Positive Habits}} \text{Lifestyle Transformation}$$

Transform behavioral patterns by cultivating positive habits, leading to a holistic lifestyle transformation.

### 14.3.8  Cognitive Agility Formula:

$$\text{Adaptive Thinking} \xrightarrow{\text{Cognitive Flexibility}} \text{Problem-Solving Mastery}$$

Develop cognitive agility through adaptive thinking, mastering problem-solving skills and overcoming challenges.

### 14.3.9  Innovative Mindset Catalyst:

$$\text{Curiosity} \xrightarrow{\text{Creative Exploration}} \text{Innovation Unleashed}$$

Fuel curiosity through creative exploration, unleashing an innovative mindset for continuous development.

### 14.3.10  Mind-Body-Soul Alignment:

$$\text{Internal Harmony} \xrightarrow{\text{Spiritual Connection}} \text{Wholeness Achieved}$$

Attain internal harmony by nurturing spiritual connection, achieving a sense of wholeness in personal development.

Continued growth and development are integral to thriving beyond depression. Embrace these strategies to propel yourself into a journey of ongoing self-improvement and fulfillment.

## 14.4 Living Authentically

### 14.4.1 Authenticity Quotient (AQ):

$$\text{Self-Expression} \xrightarrow{\text{Genuine Actions}} \text{Authentic Living}$$

Express your true self through genuine actions, leading to an increase in your Authenticity Quotient (AQ) and fostering authentic living.

### 14.4.2 Vulnerability Formula:

$$\text{Openness} \xrightarrow{\text{Transparent Communication}} \text{Emotional Connection}$$

Cultivate openness and transparent communication to establish emotional connections, embracing vulnerability as a strength.

### 14.4.3 Values Alignment Algorithm:

$$\text{Core Values} \xrightarrow{\text{Decision-Making}} \text{Life Alignment}$$

Base decision-making on core values, creating a powerful algorithm for aligning your actions with the life you desire.

### 14.4.4 Self-Discovery Equation:

$$\text{Exploration} \xrightarrow{\text{Introspection}} \text{True Identity}$$

Engage in self-exploration through introspection, unraveling layers to discover and embrace your true identity.

### 14.4.5 Courage Catalyst:

$$\text{Fear} \xrightarrow{\text{Courageous Actions}} \text{Empowered Existence}$$

Confront fears with courageous actions, transforming fear into a catalyst for an empowered existence.

### 14.4.6　Unapologetic Authenticity Theorem:

$$\text{Unfiltered Self} \xrightarrow{\text{No Apologies}} \text{Unapologetic Living}$$

Present your unfiltered self without apologies, embodying the Unapologetic Authenticity Theorem for genuine and fearless living.

### 14.4.7　Connection Multiplier:

$$\text{Authentic Relationships} \xrightarrow{\text{Mutual Understanding}} \text{Deep Connections}$$

Forge authentic relationships through mutual understanding, exponentially multiplying the depth of your connections.

### 14.4.8　Life Narrative Transformation:

$$\text{Reframing Experiences} \xrightarrow{\text{Empowerment Story}} \text{Narrative Reshaped}$$

Reframe life experiences into an empowerment story, reshaping your narrative through the lens of authenticity.

### 14.4.9　Integrity Matrix:

$$\text{Consistency} \xrightarrow{\text{Values Adherence}} \text{Integrity Fortified}$$

Maintain consistency in values adherence, fortifying the Integrity Matrix and living a life of strengthened integrity.

Living authentically is a transformative journey. Apply these formulas and theorems to cultivate authenticity, allowing your true self to shine brightly beyond the shadows of depression.

## 14.5　Sustaining Mental Well-being

### 14.5.1　Well-being Optimization Equation:

$$\text{Positive Habits} \xrightarrow{\text{Consistency}} \text{Optimized Well-being}$$

Cultivate positive habits consistently to optimize your mental well-being, creating a formula for sustained mental health.

### 14.5.2 Stress Resilience Formula:

$$\text{Resilience Skills} \xrightarrow{\text{Adaptive Coping}} \text{Stress Resistance}$$

Develop resilience skills through adaptive coping mechanisms, enhancing your stress resistance for long-term mental well-being.

### 14.5.3 Mindful Consumption Theorem:

$$\text{Mindful Awareness} \xrightarrow{\text{Selective Consumption}} \text{Positive Influence}$$

Apply mindful awareness to selectively consume content, leveraging the Mindful Consumption Theorem for a positive impact on mental health.

### 14.5.4 Neuroplasticity Principle:

$$\text{Continuous Learning} \xrightarrow{\text{Neural Growth}} \text{Mental Agility}$$

Engage in continuous learning to stimulate neural growth, embracing the Neuroplasticity Principle for enhanced mental agility.

### 14.5.5 Emotional Equilibrium Equation:

$$\text{Self-Awareness} \xrightarrow{\text{Emotional Regulation}} \text{Emotional Equilibrium}$$

Foster self-awareness and practice emotional regulation to attain and maintain emotional equilibrium.

### 14.5.6 Cognitive Nourishment Rule:

$$\text{Positive Thoughts} \xrightarrow{\text{Cognitive Nourishment}} \text{Cognitive Well-being}$$

Cultivate positive thoughts, abiding by the Cognitive Nourishment Rule to ensure sustained cognitive well-being.

### 14.5.7 Sleep Restoration Theorem:

$$\text{Quality Sleep} \xrightarrow{\text{Restoration}} \text{Mental Revitalization}$$

Prioritize quality sleep for mental restoration, applying the Sleep Restoration Theorem to achieve mental revitalization.

### 14.5.8  Mind-Body Harmony Equation:

$$\text{Physical Exercise} \xrightarrow{\text{Mind-Body Connection}} \text{Harmonized Well-being}$$

Incorporate physical exercise for a mind-body connection, achieving a state of harmonized well-being through the Mind-Body Harmony Equation.

### 14.5.9  Social Support Multiplier:

$$\text{Positive Relationships} \xrightarrow{\text{Reciprocal Support}} \text{Amplified Well-being}$$

Cultivate positive relationships with reciprocal support, multiplying the impact on your well-being through the Social Support Multiplier.

Sustaining mental well-being is a continual process. Apply these formulas and theorems consistently to foster a resilient and thriving mental state beyond the challenges of depression.

## 14.6    Creating a Legacy of Resilience

### 14.6.1  Resilience Inheritance Formula:

$$\text{Parental Resilience} \xrightarrow{\text{Modeling}} \text{Resilient Offspring}$$

By embodying and modeling resilience, parents pass on a legacy of resilience to their children through the Resilience Inheritance Formula.

### 14.6.2  Educational Amplification Theorem:

$$\text{Resilience Education} \xrightarrow{\text{Generational Impact}} \text{Amplified Resilience}$$

Embed resilience education to create a generational impact, applying the Educational Amplification Theorem for amplified resilience across communities.

### 14.6.3  Community Resilience Integration:

$$\text{Individual Resilience} \xrightarrow{\text{Community Support}} \text{Collective Resilience}$$

Individual resilience, when supported by community efforts, integrates into collective resilience, forming a robust foundation for society.

### 14.6.4 Innovation Catalyst Equation:

$$\text{Resilience Mindset} \xrightarrow{\text{Innovative Solutions}} \text{Societal Advancement}$$

A resilience mindset catalyzes innovative solutions, propelling societal advancement through the Innovation Catalyst Equation.

### 14.6.5 Adaptability Quotient (AQ) Maximization:

$$\text{Adaptive Skills} \xrightarrow{\text{Continuous Enhancement}} \text{Maximized AQ}$$

Continuous enhancement of adaptive skills maximizes the Adaptability Quotient (AQ), ensuring sustained resilience in the face of evolving challenges.

### 14.6.6 Environmental Resilience Synergy:

$$\text{Individual Actions} \xrightarrow{\text{Environmental Stewardship}} \text{Planetary Resilience}$$

Individual actions, focused on environmental stewardship, synergize to contribute to planetary resilience through the Environmental Resilience Synergy.

### 14.6.7 Technological Resilience Augmentation:

$$\text{Resilient Technologies} \xrightarrow{\text{Strategic Integration}} \text{Technological Resilience}$$

Strategically integrating resilient technologies augments technological resilience, creating a legacy of resilience in the technological landscape.

### 14.6.8 Cultural Resilience Fusion:

$$\text{Cultural Heritage} \xrightarrow{\text{Resilience Integration}} \text{Fused Cultural Resilience}$$

Integrating resilience into cultural heritage results in a fused cultural resilience, enriching societal fabric through the Cultural Resilience Fusion.

Creating a legacy of resilience involves a multi-faceted approach. Implement these formulas and theorems to establish a lasting impact on resilience across generations, communities, and the world.

# 14.7    Inspiring Others

### 14.7.1    Influence Amplification Principle:

$$\text{Individual Inspiration} \xrightarrow{\text{Shared Stories}} \text{Collective Motivation}$$

Individual inspiration, shared through compelling stories, amplifies into collective motivation, leveraging the Influence Amplification Principle.

### 14.7.2    Positivity Propagation Formula:

$$\text{Positive Actions} \xrightarrow{\text{Social Ripple Effect}} \text{Inspired Communities}$$

Engaging in positive actions initiates a social ripple effect, leading to inspired communities, following the Positivity Propagation Formula.

### 14.7.3    Motivational Quotient (MQ) Enhancement:

$$\text{Authentic Motivation} \xrightarrow{\text{Empathetic Connection}} \text{Heightened MQ}$$

Creating authentic motivation with empathetic connections enhances the Motivational Quotient (MQ), fostering a heightened motivational environment.

### 14.7.4    Leadership Catalysis Equation:

$$\text{Inspirational Leadership} \xrightarrow{\text{Empowerment}} \text{Catalyzed Inspiration}$$

Inspirational leadership, driven by empowerment, catalyzes inspiration through the Leadership Catalysis Equation.

### 14.7.5    Modeling Resilience Theorem:

$$\text{Resilient Living} \xrightarrow{\text{Observational Learning}} \text{Inspired Resilience}$$

Living resiliently, observed through observational learning, transforms into inspired resilience, following the Modeling Resilience Theorem.

### 14.7.6  Empowerment Dynamics:

$$\text{Empowering Actions} \xrightarrow{\text{Self-Efficacy}} \text{Inspired Self-Belief}$$

Empowering actions foster self-efficacy, leading to inspired self-belief through the Empowerment Dynamics.

### 14.7.7  Emotional Upliftment Formula:

$$\text{Positive Emotions} \xrightarrow{\text{Shared Expressions}} \text{Uplifted Spirits}$$

Sharing positive emotions through expressive means results in uplifted spirits, adhering to the Emotional Upliftment Formula.

### 14.7.8  Collaborative Synergy Theorem:

$$\text{Collaborative Efforts} \xrightarrow{\text{Shared Goals}} \text{Inspired Synergy}$$

Collaborative efforts, united by shared goals, yield inspired synergy as per the Collaborative Synergy Theorem.

Inspiring others involves understanding the dynamics of influence, motivation, and shared experiences. Apply these principles to create a positive impact on individuals and communities.

www.ingramcontent.com/pod-product-compliance
Lightning Source LLC
Chambersburg PA
CBHW082336270726
48658CB00017B/2872